P9-CDK-668

The Yellow World

The
Yellow World

How Fighting for My Life
Taught Me How to Live

ALBERT ESPINOSA

BALLANTINE BOOKS

NEW YORK

A Ballantine Books Trade Paperback Original

Translation copyright © 2012 by James Womack

All rights reserved.

Published in the United States by Ballantine Books, an imprint of
Random House, a division of Random House LLC,
a Penguin Random House Company, New York.

BALLANTINE and the HOUSE colophon are registered
trademarks of Random House LLC.

Originally published in Spain as *El Mundo Amarillo* by
Random House Mondadori, S.A., in 2008, copyright © 2008 by
Albert Espinosa, afterword copyright © 2008 by Eloy Azorín.
This English translation was originally published in the
United Kingdom by Particular Books in 2012.

Grateful acknowledgment is made to the Estate of Gabriel Celaya
for permission to reprint "Autobiography" by Gabriel Celaya.
Reprinted by permission of the Estate of Gabriel Celaya.

LIBRARY OF CONGRESS CATALOGING-IN-PUBLICATION DATA
Espinosa, Albert.
[Mundo amarillo. English]
The yellow world: how fighting for my life taught me
how to live / Albert Espinosa.
pages cm
ISBN 978-0-345-53812-3
eBook ISBN 978-0-345-53811-6
1. Espinosa, Albert—Health. 2. Espinosa, Albert—Childhood
and youth. 3. Espinosa, Albert—Philosophy. 4. Cancer—
Patients—Biography. 5. Cancer—Psychological aspects.
6. Self-actualization (Psychology) I. Title.
RC265.6.E76A3 2014
362.19699'40092—dc23   2014029594

Printed in the United States of America on acid-free paper

2 4 6 8 9 7 5 3 1

Book design by Dana Leigh Blanchette
Title-page and part-title image: © iStockphoto.com

Contents

Living...

The Yellows

And Relax...

The Yellow End

Introduction

My Inspiration

Gabriel Celaya was an engineer and a poet. I am an engineer and a scriptwriter. We're both left-handed. There's something about his poem "Autobiography" that goes right through me, brings a lump to my throat. I think it's because he creates his own world in this poem. His own world, Celaya world. There's nothing that affects me more than people who create their own worlds.

And this poem is built out of prohibitions, prohibitions that go to make up a life. Prohibitions that marked Celaya's life. Somehow, if we can get rid of these prohibitions we will find his life, what he thinks his life should be. He has to use so much "no" to get rid of what he doesn't want and leave us with a great heap of "yes." I like this way of looking at life.

Just like Celaya does in "Autobiography," I want to divide this book into "Beginning," "Carrying On," "Living," and

"Dying." That's four blocks that, just as he says, add up to
make anybody's life.

If you don't know the poem, here you go:

AUTOBIOGRAPHY

Don't hold the knife in your left hand.
Don't put your elbows on the table.
Fold your napkin properly.
That's the beginning.

Tell me the square root of three thousand three hundred
   and thirteen.
Where is Tanganyika? What year was Cervantes born?
I'll give you an F if you talk to your classmate.
That's how it carries on.

Do you think it's right that an engineer should write poetry?
Culture is an ornament; business is business.
If you stay with that girl you're not welcome in our house.
That's living.

Don't be so crazy. Best behavior. Stand up straight.
Don't drink. Don't smoke. Don't cough. Don't breathe.
Yes, don't breathe! Say no to every "no"
And relax: die.

                         —Gabriel Celaya

Author's Note

Why write this book?

The Yellow World is an autobiography. It is about my life when I was very young. I had cancer from the age of fourteen to twenty-four, and during those ten years I lost a leg, a lung, and part of my liver, but it was also a happy time for me. In *The Yellow World* I do not talk about cancer, I talk about what I *learned* from cancer, and everything it taught me about everyday life.

I was then inspired by this book to write a television series called *Polseres vermelles,* or *Red Band Society. Polseres vermelles* aired first in Spain, and then Italy, and perhaps the most incredible thing about this has not been the number of awards it has won or the audience it has found, but rather that Steven Spielberg bought the rights to the series for the Fox television network in the United States, with the adaptation to be done by Margaret Nagle. I have always thought that if you believe in dreams, they will come true. I've had the good fortune to have gone from a small hospital room to the big screen.

In *Red Band Society,* the world I call the yellow world, which I will go on to describe in this book, is brought to life in a very beautiful and poetic way. It's like seeing part of the book transformed and expanded. It was an honor to create and write the show in Spain, and it has been an even greater honor to be able to visit the beginning of the shooting of *Red Band Society* and know that it is in such good hands in the United States. Steven Spielberg, Margaret Nagle, Charlie

Andrews, Darryl Frank, Justin Falvey, Sergio Aguero, and everyone else involved will, I'm sure, take the series a long way.

The day Charlie Rowe, the actor playing the lead character in *Red Band Society*, had his head shaved to prepare for his role, I gave him the casino chip my hospital nurse had given me a long time ago—a charm that, according to my nurse, brings good luck to the bearer. To me, the chip has its own yellow soul and reflects the virtues of Leo, the character Charlie is to play. Leo embodies my own life, my own struggle, and someone you'll read a lot about from this page onward. I get very emotional every time I see the drama advertised as "an amazing real story." It's a great honor that the "real story" is my own story, and that it will be shared with so many people in a new way.

Back to the book. *The Yellow World* is a positive creation that is full of humor and the desire to live. Often when I walk through the streets wearing shorts, people pretend not to look at my artificial leg, but two seconds after passing me they turn around to stare at it, but I always turn as well and catch them staring. And I sometimes ask them, "Instead of staring at it, why don't you just ask me about what is clearly a very important part of my life?"

I was thirteen years old when I lost my leg, but I was lucky enough to give it a farewell party (more on that later). Aside from the party, one of the good things about losing my leg was when they asked me if I wanted to leave my leg to science. I wanted to, but for some reason science wasn't interested in it, so I ended up burying it instead. And that lets me say—and probably I am the only one here who can say it with complete confidence—that I literally have one foot in the grave.

I always say that humor helps explain everything better. And I have discovered there is humor to be found in most situations, if we choose to look for it. For example, people always think that artificial legs, like the one I have, are made of wood, like a pirate's. But I wear an electronic leg, and I find myself with the same problem that everyone with an electronic artificial leg faces: You have to recharge it at night. So in hotels where there is only one electrical outlet, I have to decide whether to recharge my laptop, my cellphone, or my artificial leg!

When we were in the hospital, the only day that we behaved like really sick kids was Christmas Day. We all knew that was the day the local soccer team would come to visit us, and they always gave a signed ball to the kid who appeared to be the sickest. So that day we all stayed in our beds with our blankets pulled up to our chins, trying to look as weak as possible. I think my greatest achievement was not beating four types of cancer; it was putting on the world's sickest face so that star player Gary Lineker gave me a soccer ball.

So, as you see, this yellow world is full of this happiness. And I've always believed that it has something to do with the lives that live on inside of me. What happened was that all of us kids who had cancer—the ones affectionately nicknamed the Eggheads—had a pact, a life pact: We'd share out the lives of the ones who died. It was an unforgettable pact, a beautiful one—we wanted to live on somehow in the others, to help them fight against cancer. And we believed that our friends who had died had weakened the cancer a little and made it easier for those of us who survived to win the battle, so it was up to us to live out their hopes and dreams.

During my ten years that I was in the hospital, when we shared out all the lives that had been lost, my share came to 3.7 lives—so with my own, that makes a total of 4.7. I'll never forget those 3.7 lives and will try always to do them justice. If it sometimes seems complicated to live your own life, imagine the responsibility involved in living 4.7 of them! 4.7 people wrote this book—4.7 lives inside me that tell you that *The Yellow World* is my favorite of all my books, and that it is an honor and gives me great happiness that it has been translated into English. I know that you will take care of this world, and that you will make it very yellow.

I hope this book will link us as yellow ones. If you have any suggestions, wishes, or you are looking for anything, you'll find me at albertespinosa23@yahoo.es.

—Albert Espinosa
July–September 2014

Beginning . . .

The Yellow World

Don't hold the knife in your left hand.
Don't put your elbows on the table.
Fold your napkin properly.
That's the beginning.

—Gabriel Celaya

Where Were You Born?

Well, I was born from cancer. I like the word *cancer*. I even like the word *tumor*. It might sound creepy but it's just that my life has been connected to these two words. And I've never felt anything horrible about saying *cancer* or *tumor* or *osteosarcoma*. I grew up with these words and I like to say them out loud, to shout them at the top of my voice. I think that until you say them, make them part of your life, then it's difficult for you to accept them.

That's why I need to speak about cancer in this first chapter, because later in the book I'm going to explain the lessons that cancer taught me to survive my life. So I'll start off by talking about it and how it affected me.

I was fourteen years old when I had to go to the hospital for the first time. I had an osteosarcoma in my left leg. I left school, left my home, and started my life in the hospital.

I had cancer for ten years, from the ages of fourteen to twenty-four. This doesn't mean that I spent ten years in the hospital but that for ten years I was going to various different hospitals to get treated for four cancers: leg, leg (same leg both times), lung, and liver.

En route I left behind one leg, one lung, and a chunk of my liver. But I have to say that, at the time, I was happy when I had cancer. I remember it as one of the best times of my life.

It might be a shock to see these two words next to each other: *happy* and *cancer*. But that's how it was. The cancer might have taken material things away from me, but it taught me lots of other things that I would never have found out by myself.

What can cancer give you? I think the list is endless: You find out who you are, you find out what sort of people you live with, you discover your limits . . . above all you lose your fear of death. Maybe this last is the most valuable thing.

One day I was cured. I was twenty-four and they told me that I didn't have to go back to the hospital. I was scared stiff. It was weird. The thing I knew how to do best of all was to fight against cancer and now they told me that I was cured. This weirdness, this stupor, lasted for six hours, then I went mad with joy; not to go back to the hospital, not to have any more X-rays (I think I'd had more than two hundred and fifty), no more blood tests, no more tests of any kind. It was a dream come true. It was completely unbelievable.

I thought that in a few months I'd forget all about cancer. I'd have a "normal life." Cancer would just be a stage I'd gone through. But instead (I've never forgotten it), something strange happened. I never imagined how much the lessons of cancer would help me in my daily life.

It's the great gift that cancer has given me: lessons (you

have to call them something, although maybe I prefer the word *discoveries*) that help my life to be easier, happier.

What I will explain in this book is nothing more than how to apply to your day-to-day life the lessons I learned from cancer. Yes, exactly, now that I think of it, that's what this book could be called: *How to Use Cancer to Get Through Life*. Maybe that'll end up being the book's subtitle. It sounds odd, it sounds just the opposite of most of the books that get written about cancer, but that's just how it is. Life is paradoxical (I love contradictions). I want to make it clear that this book is a collection of everything I learned from cancer and also of the discoveries that my friends who were also fighting this illness showed me.

Well, that's the story of cancer and me up till now. I like how I've summed it up; I'm happy with it. The story has begun. Now let's carry on with the yellow world.

What Is the Yellow World?

This is something you've probably been asking yourself ever since you bought this yellow book (at least, I imagine it as being yellow; we'll see what happens when it gets published— maybe the cover will end up being red, or orange, or a kind of brownish gray).

The yellow world is the name I've given to a way of living, of seeing life, of nourishing yourself with the lessons that you learn from good moments as well as bad ones. The yellow world is made out of discoveries, above all, yellow discoveries, which are those that give it its name. But don't worry; we'll get there in a bit. No hurry.

What I can tell you from the beginning is that this is a universe with no rules. Most worlds are controlled by a set of rules, but the yellow world has no rules. I don't like rules, so I wouldn't like my world to have them. It'd be a bit odd. And I don't think that rules are necessary; they're useless, they exist just to be jumped over, gotten around, bypassed. I don't think that anything they tell you is sacred actually is. I don't think that anything they tell you is correct actually is. Everything has a flip side; everything can be seen from lots of different points of view.

I have always believed that the yellow world is the world we actually live in. The world we see in movies, the world of cinema, is one created out of false ideas, and we end up thinking that the world is really like that. They show you what love is like, and then you fall in love and it's not like it is in the movies. They show you what sex is like, and then you have sex and it's also not like how it is in the movies. They even show you what breakups are like. How many times have people met their boyfriend or girlfriend in a bar and tried to break up like they do in the movies? It doesn't work. It doesn't work because on film they can get it over and done with in five minutes, but it actually takes you six hours and in the end you don't break up but promise to get married or have a child.

And I don't believe in these labels that they say define various generations. I don't think I'm part of Generation X, or Generation iPod, and I'm definitely not part of any metrosexual or übersexual generation.

What am I? Yellow (something individual that isn't part of any collective). I'm yellow, I'm somebody's yellow. But like I said, we'll get there in a bit.

So, there aren't any labels, any rules, any norms of behavior. I suppose you're probably asking how I'm going to put this book, and this world, in order; how I'm going to get my thoughts straight. Well, I'm going to make a list. I believe in lists; I like lists. I'm an engineer; I became one because I like numbers, and if you like numbers then you like lists.

From here on in, everything you read is a big list. A list of concepts, a list of ideas, a list of feelings, a happy list. A list of discoveries that I made and that make up what I think of as my world.

They're short discoveries that I set out in short chapters. They're little elements that let us see the world in a different way. Don't be afraid of living in the yellow world. All you have to do is believe in it.

I've got one maxim: Trust your dreams and they'll come true. *Trust* and *true* are very similar words, and they are similar because they are actually close to each other, really very close. So close that if you do trust something, it will come true.

Trust it. . . .

And now we'll go straight to the big section where I've put all these discoveries: *how to live* . . . Here are the experiences of cancer related to life, which form the elements you can combine to create your yellow world.

It's a list of twenty-three points that you should connect with lines, connect conceptually in your mind: Do this and a way of living will appear. A yellow world.

Every point, every discovery, is connected with one of the phrases I heard during my hospital life. They're things people said to me while I was ill and that had such an effect on me that I've never forgotten them. They're like extracts from a poem, or the beginnings of songs, sentiments that will always smell of chemotherapy, or bandages, or waiting for visits or roommates in their blue pajamas. Sometimes it's words that show you the way. A few words can come together and provoke an idea. Sometimes the most important phrases are those we give the least importance.

So come in, and trust this, a little. Believe what I'm saying, but keep your eyes open. Everything can be questioned, debated. The guy who's telling you this is me, Albert. Agnostic. Apolitical. Yellow.

Carrying On . . .

List of Discoveries to Make Your World Yellow

(Lessons from Cancer Applied to Life)

Tell me the square root of three thousand three hundred
    and thirteen.
Where is Tanganyika? What year was Cervantes born?
I'll give you an F if you talk to your classmate.
That's how it carries on.

—Gabriel Celaya

1

Losses are positive

Give your leg a goodbye party. Invite all the people who have some connection to your leg and give it a great send-off. Hasn't it supported you all your life? Well, support it now that it's walking away.

—my traumatologist,
the day before they cut off my leg

Losses are positive. I know that's a hard thing to believe, but losses are positive. We have to learn how to lose things. You need to know that whatever you win, sooner or later, you'll end up losing.

In the hospital they taught us to accept loss, but rather than putting the emphasis on accepting, they put it on loss. Accepting something is only a matter of time; losing something is a question of principles.

Years ago, whenever someone died, his close family would go through a period of mourning: They would wear black, suffer, and stay at home. The mourning period gave them time to think about the loss, to live for the loss.

We've gone from mourning to nothing. Now when someone dies they tell you in the funeral home that you've got to get over it. You break up with your partner and people tell you that you'll be going out with someone else in a couple of weeks. But what about the mourning? Where's the mourning gone, the thinking about the loss, about what loss means?

Cancer took a lot away from me: parts of my body, mobility, experiences, years of school . . . But what I felt most of all was probably the loss of my leg. I remember that the day before they cut it off my doctor said to me: "Give your leg a goodbye party. Invite all the people who have some connection to your leg and give it a great send-off. Hasn't it supported you all your life? Well, support it now that it's walking away."

I was fifteen and I hadn't organized a party to lose my virginity (I'd have liked that) but I was organizing a party to lose my leg. I remember as if it were only this morning how I phoned people who were connected with the leg (it was a bit tough, it wasn't easy to get people to come). After going over things a lot in my head and talking about hundreds of things, I ended up saying to them: "I'm inviting you to the goodbye party for my leg; you don't have to bring anything. And come on foot." I thought it was important to mention that just to stop things from being awkward. Some genius decided to give us a sense of humor, the cure for all our worries. . . . A strange ability: to be able to turn everything upside down and laugh at it.

The people I invited to this strange party were those who

had had some kind of relationship with my leg: a goalkeeper who let in forty-five goals from me in one match (well, okay, only one, but I invited him anyway), a girl I played footsie with under the table, one of my uncles, who took me hiking (because of the cramps I'd gotten in my legs, and anyway I couldn't think of many more people to invite), and a friend who had a dog that bit me when I was ten. The worst of it was that the dog came and tried to bite me again.

It was a great party. I think it was the best party I've ever given, and definitely the most original. Everyone was a bit shy at the beginning, but we started bit by bit to talk about the leg. Everyone told stories about it. They touched it one last time. It was a night I'll never forget.

When the night came to an end and dawn was breaking, a few hours before I went into surgery, I suddenly thought of the best possible finishing touch: one last dance. I asked a nurse to dance with me and she said yes. I didn't have any music but my roommate had lots of Antonio Machín CDs (he was a big fan of Machín, and even called himself "El Manisero"*). I put on the CD he lent me and out came "Wait for Me in Heaven." There was no more suitable song for this moment, for the last moment. I danced maybe a dozen times with the nurse. My last dozen dances. I danced so much! All I really wanted was not to hear anything, for Machín to melt magically with my mind, become nothing more than a repetitive noise, the perfect soundtrack. Don't you like it when a piece of music is repeated so many times that you don't

---

* Antonio Machín (1903–77): Cuban singer, most famous for "El Manisero" ("The Peanut Vendor"), the first Cuban song to be a hit in the U.S.

hear the words, the individual sounds? This music, these words, they end up being just like the wind, something that's there, that you notice, that you don't need to listen to, just feel.

The next day they cut my leg off. But I wasn't sad; I'd said goodbye to it, I'd cried, I'd laughed. Without realizing, I'd had my mourning period. I'd spoken about the loss without any hang-ups and I'd turned it into a gain.

I like to think that I haven't actually lost a leg but gained a stump. Along with a list of leg-related memories:

1. A wonderful goodbye party. (How many people can say that they've had a party that cool?)
2. The memory of my second set of baby steps (you forget about the first ones, but you never forget your second set, the first baby steps with your mechanical leg).
3. Also, as I mentioned earlier, because I buried my leg, I'm one of the few people in this world who can literally say that they've got one foot in the grave. I always like to think that I'm one of the lucky ones, to be able to say that.

Of course losses are positive. Cancer taught me this. But this is something that can be brought across into the noncancerous world. We suffer losses every day: sometimes important ones that upset us; sometimes smaller ones that only worry us. It's not like losing a leg, but the technique for getting over them is the same as I learned in the hospital.

If, when you lose something, you convince yourself that

you aren't losing it, then you've beaten the loss. Let it go: Mourn for a bit if you need to. The steps are as follows:

1. Focus on the loss; think about it.
2. Suffer with it. Call the people connected with the loss, ask their advice.
3. Cry. (Our eyes are our private and public windshield wipers.)
4. Look for what you can gain from the loss (take your time).
5. In a few days you'll feel better. You'll see what you've gained. But remember that you can lose this feeling as well.

Does it work? Of course. I never had a phantom limb. A phantom limb is when you still feel the leg even when you don't have it anymore. I think that I don't have one because, even without knowing, I gave the real leg such a good send-off that even its ghost went away.

The first discovery of the yellow world: Losses are positive. Don't let anyone tell you any different.

Sometimes the losses will be small; other times they'll be big. But if you get used to understanding them, to facing up to them, in the end you'll realize that they don't really exist. Every loss is a gain.

2

The word *pain* doesn't exist

What if injections don't actually hurt? What if what happens is that we react to pain like they show us in the movies without noticing if we really feel it? What if pain doesn't actually exist?

—David, a real Egghead,
who gave me 60 percent of his life

There's no such thing as pain. This was the phrase that I heard people using most often with the Eggheads while I was in the hospital. The Eggheads was the name that some of the doctors and nurses used for us, on account of our lack of hair. It normally means someone really bright, but I like it when words do their own thing, when mistakes create different sorts of ideas. We liked the name: It made us feel part of a gang, made us feel young, strong, and healthy. Sometimes labels work so well that they make you feel better. . . .

In the Eggheads, just like in any gang with any pride, we

had a couple of slogans that we liked to shout: "I've only got one leg, but I'm not lame." That made us feel proud of ourselves. The second-most popular: "There's no such thing as pain." Because we shouted it so much, threw this statement out to the world, eventually the pain itself went away.

There is something called the pain threshold, the moment when you start to notice pain; it's the doorway into pain, the moment when your brain thinks that something is going to make it hurt. The pain threshold is half a centimeter away from actual pain. Yes, it is possible to measure it. I think it must be because I'm an engineer that I use numbers to judge feelings, people, and pain. Sometimes I think that it's the mixture of engineering and cancer that's made me like this.

So little by little, we stopped noticing pain. First of all it was the pain of the chemo injections; it always hurts when they give you an injection. But we found out that the pain came from thinking that it existed. "What if injections don't actually hurt? What if what happens is that we react to pain like they show us in the movies without noticing if we really feel it? What if pain doesn't actually exist?"

All of these ideas came from the cleverest of the Eggheads. He'd had cancer since he was seven, and when he came up with this he was fifteen. For me he was and always will be a mirror in which I see myself. He pulled us together; he talked to us; you could almost say that he taught us; and certainly he could always convince us of anything.

When I heard him say that pain could disappear if we just refused to believe it existed, I thought this was an incredibly stupid idea, and when he spoke to me about the pain threshold I didn't understand anything.

But one day in a chemo session (and they gave me more than eighty-three), I decided to believe what he'd told me. I looked at the needle, I looked at my skin, and I didn't introduce the third variable. It didn't form a part of the pain equation. I didn't think that pain was inevitable. It was just a needle that came close to my skin, went through my skin, and took some blood. It was like being caressed, a strange, different kind of caress. Iron stroking the flesh.

And mysteriously it happened, just like that: For the first time I didn't notice any pain. I just felt this strange caress. That day the nurse needed to stick the needle in twelve times to find a vein, because with chemo the veins hide away and get more and more difficult to find. I didn't complain a single time, because it was magic, almost poetic, to think about this sensation. It wasn't pain; it was something that didn't have a name but which didn't resemble pain at all.

That was the day when I discovered that *pain* is a word that has no real value; it's just like *fear*. They're two words that frighten you, that provoke pain and fear. But when the word doesn't exist, the thing it tries to define doesn't exist, either.

I think that what this great Egghead, who gave me 60 percent of his life (the best 60 percent I've got), wanted to say was that the word *pain* doesn't exist; just that, that it doesn't exist as a word, as a concept. You have to work out what's happening to you (like I did with the injection) and not think that it's the same as feeling pain. You have to test it, taste it, and decide what it is that you're feeling. I insist that often "pain" will be pleasure, "pain" will be enjoyable, "pain" will be poetic.

In the seven years afterward that I had cancer I never felt any pain, because the majority of cancer cases (apart from 10 or 12 percent) are not painful. It's movies that have turned it into something painful. It's difficult for me to think of a movie in which someone with cancer doesn't cry from pain, or vomit, or die, or take huge amounts of morphine. They always show the same things: pain and death.

When I wrote *4th Floor** it was, above all, because I wanted to write a positive movie, a realistic one, one that would deal with the issue properly and show what the lives of people with cancer are really like. How they live through all this "false" pain that the movies show. How they fight and how they die, yes, but how not everything revolves around vomit, pain, and death.

When I got better I thought that I'd forget this lesson, but actually it was the first one I remembered. There is a lot of pain outside of the hospital and hospital life, pain that isn't medical, that doesn't have anything to do with injections or surgical operations. There's pain that comes from other people, people who inflict pain whether willingly or unwillingly.

And it was in my cancer-free life that I really felt pain: pain from love, from sadness, from pride, in my work. This was when I remembered that pain doesn't exist; the word *pain* doesn't exist. When I started to go back to thinking about what I really felt when these things happened to me, I realized that sometimes it was nostalgia, sometimes it was

---

* *4th Floor* (*Planta 4ª*, directed by Antonio Mercero, 2003): a comedy-drama about four teenage long-term patients in the cancer wing of a Spanish hospital.

defenselessness, sometimes unease, and sometimes loneliness. But it wasn't pain.

When I was a boy, when I learned in the hospital that pain doesn't exist, I felt, at the age of fourteen, like a superhero whose power was never to feel pain.

I had a friend who said: "It's like you're made out of iron; you never notice when something pricks you." Now that I'm older I realize that I still get pricked all the time: sometimes three or four pricks all at once in different places, sometimes only once, right in the heart. The secret is not to be unfeeling or made of iron, but to allow yourself to be penetrated, to be touched, and then to rename whatever it is you feel.

The list is easy. The discovery is easy: The word *pain* doesn't exist. Step by step . . .

1. Think of words whenever you think of *pain*. Look for five or six that define what you're feeling, but don't let any of them be *pain*.
2. When you've got them, think of the one that best defines whatever you're feeling; this is your "pain." This is the word that defines what you're feeling.
3. Get rid of the word *pain* and substitute the new word. Stop feeling "pain" and feel this new definition as strongly as possible. Feel this sentiment.

It might seem impossible for this to work, but with time you'll control it and realize that pain doesn't exist. Physical pain, an aching heart—all of these really conceal other sensations, other feelings. And these can be overcome. When you know what you're feeling, it's easier to get over it.

3

The energy that appears after thirty minutes is what you need to solve a problem

Whatever you do, don't open the envelope with the results of the X-ray.
—doctor to patient

Let's open it right away.
—patient to family
when he gets the envelope

Very often in the hospital we had to get test results. There's no moment of greater tension than when you've got the envelope with the CAT scan or the X-ray results in your hand.

Over the course of ten years, this situation repeated itself lots of times. They would give you the X-rays and the envelope with the results and tell you again and again that you weren't to open it, that you should give it to the doctor.

There was normally about two weeks between getting the results and the doctor's appointment. Two weeks is a long time to keep an envelope closed when what's inside it might tell you that there's been a relapse, that the cancer has returned in some part of your body. (That's the shortest way to put it: A relapse means you can definitely say you've got cancer again.)

All of my friends in the hospital, all of them, opened their envelopes. Of course they did. How can you think that it would be possible to keep something so important closed for two weeks?

I've recently been giving some feedback to doctors about how they should treat patients and I always tell them that this is the first thing they've got to change: It's such an old-fashioned procedure. The doctors always smile as if they are saying we know you'll open it. It's like an unwritten pact: You'll open it, you'll read it, you'll stick the flap back down, and then we'll pretend we don't notice. I've always been shocked by this sort of pact; I don't know why everyone knows things and then pretends that they don't. It doesn't make any sense.

Anyway, the important thing is not the envelope but what's in the envelope. The problem is how to face an important piece of news, one that could change your life. We learned how to do it in the hospital; we learned by making mistakes, which is how you learn almost anything in this life.

To begin with, we would open the envelope frantically, right there in the hospital, two minutes after it was handed over. I remember a few images from the hospital corridor: my father, my mother, and me leaning over the sheet of paper, reading (maybe better to say devouring) what was written on it.

A little bit later we realized that it wasn't a good idea to open it in the hospital: You shouldn't give or get bad news in a place where you have spent or are going to spend a lot of time. You have to find somewhere neutral. So we would open the envelope in restaurants (ones that we were going to for the first time), in unknown streets (whose names we later forgot), or in the metro. But we were still making a mistake: We never let more than fifteen minutes pass from getting the envelope to opening it. Without realizing, we looked for nearby restaurants, streets, or metro stations. We had an urgent need to know what was in the envelope, as if something were burning us from the inside.

With time, after they had given us forty or fifty envelopes, we discovered the perfect method. There's no doubt that you can become a professional even when it comes to reading medical diagnoses: All you need to do is repeat the action over and over again until it doesn't seem like you're repeating it.

The perfect method:

1. Take the envelope calmly, put it away, and take it home without thinking about it. . . .
2. Wait for exactly half an hour without thinking about the envelope, without giving it a single second of your time. And when exactly half an hour has passed . . .
3. Go to a calm place and open it. This half hour is all the time your body needs to calm down and all the time your mind needs to become serene; it's as if all your anxiety disappears. The best thing about this is that when you react to the results, they're half an hour older

as well. It's as if they were old news and this takes away their strength and gives you power.

I know this might seem strange. Why half an hour and not an hour? Why not ten minutes? Are these thirty minutes that important? Yes, they are. I think that through receiving so many pieces of important news, I've discovered that there's something in us that wants to know the news immediately, and this something blinds us. It's like a passion that vanishes after exactly thirty minutes and activates other energies in us, energies that also want to know what's happened but that are capable of looking for solutions. These energies are a form of anxiety but a form with a different aim, anxiety that fights, that resolves problems.

When I stopped going to the hospital I thought that I would never be faced with dilemmas as powerful as the ones I had about the X-rays. And that's how it was, but I've found a way of adapting my thirty-minute theory to real life.

I often receive an email that I know is important; I see it pop up in my inbox but I don't open it. I look at it, still up there with its title in bold, but I don't open it. I wait for thirty minutes. I relax, I let my anxiety change, and then I open it.

It's great, and it works. And whether it's good or bad news that you're getting, you've let half an hour pass and your response isn't hasty, the result of an immediate reaction. It's as if you've spent half an hour deciding what to write. You can do the same with text messages, and lots of other things as well.

This is also useful for when you need to discuss something with someone, especially when it comes to choosing the time and the place you speak to them.

I always follow the thirty-minute rule and sometimes, I must admit, I stretch it as far as forty or even as many as forty-three minutes. It's a way of stretching time, of being the lord and master of your anxieties and your responses.

4

Ask five good questions every day

Take an exercise book and write; write down every-
thing you don't understand.

—my doctor,
the day he told me I had cancer

This was the first piece of advice my doctor gave me when I got to the hospital. In fact, what he did was give me an exercise book and tell me to write down everything I didn't understand.

Then he explained to me everything that would happen to me, cancerously speaking, over the next five years. It was amazing; he got it almost all right. Sometimes I dream about this moment and imagine what would have happened if, instead of talking to me about cancer, he had spoken about my life. He could have predicted my life for the next five or ten years. Who I would fall in love with, what I would end up studying. That would have been even more amazing.

But I don't want to minimize the importance of what he said, because it turned out as he predicted. He spoke to me about biopsies, tumors, osteosarcomas, relapses. My parents listened to him and I took notes; I kept on taking notes. It was weird, but I even felt better as I was writing things down. It was as if, by getting my questions out into the open, by writing them down, I was stripping them of their mystery, their fear, their terror.

When he'd finished, he looked at me and said: "Any questions?" I replied that I had forty-two of them. That was all I'd had time to write down. That day he answered my forty-two questions, but I came up with twenty more. The more he explained, the more questions I had, but the more of those he answered the more peaceful I felt. It was a circle, good for both him and me.

I've never doubted the fact that possessing information is fundamental for everything in life. You can't fight against cancer if you don't know what you're up against. First know who your enemy is, then find out everything about him and only then fight against him.

I think that the best thing about the time I had cancer was that they always gave me answers. Answers cure you; answers help you. Asking questions makes you feel alive. When they give you answers it means that they trust you'll know what to do with the information.

But you don't just have questions when you feel ill. Life itself generates a huge number of questions. When I left the hospital I started to ask myself questions. I'd left school at the age of fifteen and didn't get back to my education until I went to college. I had hundreds of questions. This was when

I decided to buy myself a yellow notebook (I didn't know why I chose that color, but I realize now). I started to write down questions and to decide who to ask about them.

It was easy in the hospital:

1. Difficult questions to the doctor.
2. Halfway difficult ones to the nurse.
3. Easy ones (or the most complicated ones) to the orderlies and my roommates.

But in life itself not everything is so clear. So I would write down the question, the problem I wanted to solve, and the person I should ask about it. I really recommend you do this; you'll start off by thinking that it's ridiculous to write down silly questions and the people who you think might have the answers. But as you start to get answers you'll realize that the method is very effective, and you'll become an addict of your little notebook.

I've used this method in every aspect of my life: my love life, my family life, my friendships, my yellow life (in a bit, I'll explain what the yellow life is). And it has always made me feel better.

So, it's easy:

1. Choose a color for your notebook. The color has to have something to do with you. Each of us has a color that has nothing to do with the clothes we wear. Maybe you love your blue jeans but your color might be orange. It's really easy to find your color. Look at a box

of felt-tip pens and choose one to draw with; the one you choose will be your color.

2. Buy ten notebooks. Yes, I know. It might seem that one is enough, but actually each book is for a different aspect of the world. I've always thought that people have ten different worries about the world, ten possible paths through it. So use one book per path.

3. Write down all your queries. Stupid queries: How do people manage to get their hair looking nice? Complicated queries: How can it be that people fall in love and I only think about sex? Eternal queries: Who am I? Who do I want to be? Do I really know nothing? Practical queries: How do you rent a light aircraft? How do you proceed with a divorce?

4. Look for the person who has the answers. Next to each question you should write down a possible candidate for the answer. Never leave this bit empty; put someone down, even if you don't yet know them personally, even if it's someone famous or invented or impossible.

5. Ask, absorb the answer, note down the queries that emerge, and ask again. The more queries you get answered the better you'll feel.

In the hospital they told us that it is good to drink two liters of water a day. And my doctor always added: "And ask five good questions." Don't forget it, five questions a day and two liters of water.

5

Show me how you walk and I'll show you how to laugh

It's not easy to laugh. It's not easy to breathe, either.
There aren't any schools for laughing and breathing.
Am I boring you?
—the last words I heard from the nurse who took me
to the operating room to get my leg cut off

We are born lacking things, lots of things, lots of very different things. With time we manage to cover this up in some way or another. Sometimes we do it well; sometimes we just do it as best we can. We even end up not knowing that we're missing things. The brain is so clever that sometimes it hides very basic things about us from ourselves.

We don't know how to walk, but we find out bit by bit how to walk. I've been lucky enough to have four kinds of walk:

1. My first steps, a year or so after I was born. It was a walk made up of quick steps and as I approached ado-

lescence it was becoming a bit naughty. A walk that made me laugh a lot, in lots of different strange ways.

2. Years later, my second first steps, when they gave me my first mechanical leg. It was a slightly cruder walk, more like bouncing on a spring. A walk that changed the way I was, stopped me feeling comfortable, and stopped me laughing.

3. Then they switched me over to a hydraulic leg. This gave me a walk that was more cheerful, more singsong, more like something out of a musical. It made me feel better and I started to laugh in short, glissando-like bursts. This was when I realized that laughing and walking are connected. Show me how you walk and I'll show you how you laugh. There's something in the way we walk that affects our laughter, our sense of humor.

4. Now I've got an electronic leg, and walking and laughing seem absolutely connected. The weirdest thing is when I need to charge it up at night. Sometimes I don't know whether to charge my computer, my cellphone, or my leg. I think it's a luxury to have problems like this.

There is something fundamental about walking. People don't really think about walking: "I walk like this, I've always walked like this." They think it's not going to change: If they've walked that way for thirty, forty years, why should they change now?

But what they don't realize is that change is possible. Everything depends on finding the right way to breathe, finding the most suitable way for you to breathe. Devoting a bit of time to feeling the air coming in and out of you. Once you find your way of breathing, you need to think about how this breathing can move your legs. Breathing and movement are completely related.

Little by little you'll find a way to walk. It'll be different from the one you have at the moment. It'll be a walk that's brought into existence by the way that you breathe in and out. In lots of cases it will be a walk that's so different that you won't recognize yourself in a mirror, so different that you won't think it's you walking but someone else. Little by little, if you want, you can turn this new way of walking into a new way of running. But that's something for the true initiates.

In the end you'll notice that finding a different walk, a different way of bringing your feet into contact with the ground, will cause something to be born within you. A feeling a little like happiness. This is the seed of laughter. This feeling, this sentiment, is what will transform into laughter.

Little by little, without hurrying, extract and liquefy the laughter that has arisen from this way of walking. Try out the laugh that suits you best. Listen to it, first of all in your own home, in intimate surroundings. When you've decided on one, show it to your friends, laugh with them, without being scared, without being ashamed. Let yourself go.

This is your laugh. All you have to do is exploit it to its maximum potential and, almost without your knowing it, this laugh will change who you are and how you enjoy life.

We spend minutes deciding what we want to buy in a shop, hours choosing a car, months hunting for a house. But for something that is as intimate as a laugh, something that defines our character, our essence, our being, we are usually happy with the one that comes as a default.

Remember, the list goes like this:

1. Find a way to breathe. How? By breathing: by taking in and letting out air. Think about the way of breathing that defines you. Don't think that you'll find it in a day; give yourself a week at least. Enjoy yourself.

2. Practice breathing like this as you move around. Let this new way of oxygenating yourself get all the way down to your feet. Walk fast, walk slowly, walk on tip-toe: whatever it takes. You'll end up finding your way of walking; you'll notice it when you do.

3. Walk, and enjoy the feeling of walking. Do it for half an hour. This feeling of happiness can develop into laughter. What you feel is the material that laughter is made of. Laugh, smile, and fix upon a way of emitting the sound of your happiness.

4. Practice this at home. Practice it with friends. It's a good idea to imitate the way your friends laugh. A merry-go-round of laughter is very positive.

5. Choose a laugh, and believe that this is something that defines you. Feel proud of your new acquisition and show it to people with pride. You've found a way of breathing, a way of walking, and a way of laughing. These are things that you should show off without any shame, just like a child does.

6. Renew your laugh every two years. Every two years I change my leg and I'm lucky enough that when I change the way I walk I change everything. Our lungs evolve,

they get older, but it shouldn't be these that control the way we breathe; we've got to take control and be the ones who decide how we want to oxygenate ourselves.

Breathe, walk, laugh, enjoy yourself. It's that easy. This was the advice that the nurse gave me as he took me to surgery when they were going to cut off my leg. I was thinking about the leg I was going to lose and he spoke to me about breathing, about walking, about laughing. Remember that he ended up by asking if he was boring me. Actually, I wasn't bored at all. Sometimes we are so focused on ourselves, on our own problems, that we forget that we are right at that moment on the edge of making the greatest discovery of our lives.

6

When you are sick, they keep tabs on your life, a medical record. When you are well, you should do the same: Keep a life record

The patient is cured.

—the last sentence and the last line that
my oncologist wrote on my medical record

My medical record is endless; it grew fatter day by day, month by month, year by year. The last time I went to the hospital they brought it on a cart; it was so big that they couldn't carry it.

I like the color of the file they used for the record, mostly because it's the same shade as it was on the first day. There are few things in our lives that stay the same. It's still a neutral gray color. I don't think gray is ugly; it's just got a bad reputation: gray days, gray suits . . . It's a much underappreciated color, beaten only by black. But I think it's the perfect color for a medical record because, as I see it, a record has to be distinguished, and gray is a very distinguished color.

There are letters from more than twenty doctors in my file:

1. From my oncologist (a strange job, but someone has to do it). They're the bad guys for anyone who's got cancer. Any doctor who chooses this as his specialty deserves my complete admiration.
2. From my traumatologist, who's the guy who has all the success. I'd have liked to have been a traumatologist; it seems to me the closest thing to being God.
3. From my physiotherapist . . .
4. From my radiologist . . .
5. From . . .

The list goes on. I remember when I was a kid I went to get soccer players' autographs; this is the same but with doctors, and with the added difference that instead of a single illegible scrawl there are hundreds.

The last day that I saw my file was in the oncologist's office. He wrote, "The patient is cured." Underneath it, I remember perfectly, he drew a horizontal line. The line impressed me greatly. He closed the file, put it back on the cart, and the orderly took it away. That was the last time I saw it.

I thought I wouldn't miss the file. But when I returned to normal life, I thought it would be a good idea to have one: not a medical history but a life history.

I bought a file (gray, of course) and thought about what to

put into it. I was sure that I would write a diary: Diaries are living objects and extremely recommendable. How good it is to be able to read the things that worried you two or three years ago and to realize that now you couldn't care less about them (sometimes because they're goals that you've attained, sometimes because they're things you didn't really want anyway).

But diaries are only a part of a life history; they're not enough in themselves. The pleasure of having a life history is to be able to include anything that happens in your life, every important moment, and when something stresses you out you can go to your record, open it, and calm yourself down.

You might ask if it's necessary to have this sort of control for your life. My answer is a definite "yes." Do you know why people have medical histories? Simply to note down and be sure about when a crisis occurred, how it was overcome, when the next setback occurred, what they felt when it came along, how it was sorted out. Whenever there was a problem, my doctors would always look at the medical record. I'm sure I managed to avoid loads of X-rays, blood tests, and duplicate prescriptions. Memory is so selective. . . .

The good thing about writing these things down is that it shows you how life is cyclical: Everything comes back and keeps on coming back. The problem is that our memory is very small and very forgetful. You'll be fascinated to see how your high points and low points repeat themselves, and your life history will have a solution for everything in your life.

I know what you're thinking. Don't be afraid; it won't take up too much of your time. All you need to do is write for a few minutes each day and gather together objects and things that are comparable to X-rays or the results of blood tests. These are important: There's no good record that doesn't contain evidence (in this case bits of your life). They could be bits of napkin (from the restaurant where you managed to get something you wanted), rocks from some beach (where your life took one step forward and you felt complete), or even just the ticket from the parking garage at the shopping center where you parked the day you saw the film that changed your life.

Your life record will get bigger and bigger and eventually maybe you'll need to buy a second and a third file.

If you're lucky, one day you'll die (yes, if you're lucky) and your children, your friends, your yellows (who are your yellows, you wonder? We will get to that in due time) will inherit this life history and will know what it was that made you happy, what made you feel complete. Is there anything more valuable than that they should know you better? I don't think so. This is the true reward: to open up the private boxes of the people we love and know more about them. I have so many friends with information hidden away within them, and whenever I find out something more about them I feel happier, more complete.

Here's the list for your life record:

1. Buy a file that's large, almost like a box. You get to choose the color, but I recommend gray.
2. Every day write down three or four things that have made you feel happy. Only this: Don't force yourself too much. Write: "I felt happy today."
3. Next, write down when, where, and why. Does every-

thing have to be connected to happiness? No, of course not. You can talk about nostalgia, smiles, irony. But everything has to be positive. In a medical record you don't write about anything apart from mishaps, problems, and recuperation; in a life record you should talk about life, positive, happy life. Carry out this exercise: Think about good things that have happened to you, with whom and where. Little by little you'll discover patterns. People who make you happy, places and times of day that make you feel more alive.

4. Include physical material. Whenever you can, incorporate an object that's got some relationship to the particular moment. Objects become impregnated with happiness and should be in your life record. Anything will do; all it has to do is belong to the place. But don't put in thousands and thousands of objects; you have to be selective or else your life record will end up eating your house.

5. Reread it; touch it when you feel bad and sad and also when you feel happy. At least once every six months give it a once-over; examine your life record. You'll discover things, patterns that show you how you are. Every extra 1 percent of yourself that you discover is a step further toward another state of mind.

6. Gift it: Leave it to someone when you die. Remember, it's not just for you, but also for other people, the people who love you.

I think that the day someone inherits my medical history and my life history will be a marvelous one. The person who gets them will be happy with both records. One will tell him how many leucocytes I had in October 1988, what my left leg looked like in X-rays (there's not a lot of people who know that), and, above all, will give him that final horizontal line. How beautiful a single line can be! The other record will show him why I laughed, what I got excited about, why I died. I think I'll give them to two different people. It's always good for knowledge to be shared.

7

There are seven tricks to being happy

Hey, kid, you're not sleeping, right? Listen, this is the
first one. The most important thing in life is to know
how to say no. Write it down so you won't forget.
—my first roommate, Mr. Fermín (age seventy-six),
at 5:12 in the morning

This is a piece of advice that an old man with whom I shared my first hospital room gave me. It was a six-man room; later they moved me into a two-man one. He gave me this advice very early one morning: Early mornings bring people together so much that you get the courage to confess desires and inadmissible dreams. Then the day comes and with it . . . with it . . . sometimes there comes regret.

Mr. Fermín was an impressive man: He'd had thirty different jobs, was seventy-six years old, and had a life full of incredible stories. For a kid of fourteen who was coming into the hospital for the first time, this was the mirror I wanted to reflect myself in, the future I wanted and wasn't sure I was going to be able to attain. I thought this man was really great. He was pure energy.

He always ate oranges; he loved oranges. He smelled citrusy. Over the seven nights he shared a room with me he gave me advice about how to have a good life; he gave me what he called the seven rules for being happy.

Every rule came with an explanation that lasted an hour, with lots of graphic examples. The people who studied in these life-lesson classes were a fellow Egghead from the Canary Islands with one arm and me (who would later end up with one leg). His dissertations were very enjoyable, great fun. He made us take note of everything. I think that a lot of times he thought we didn't understand anything at all. And he was right. I understood almost nothing, but those notes in my adolescent handwriting have lasted me the rest of my life.

He made us promise that we would never tell these seven rules to anyone unless we felt ourselves to be close to death. Both of us promised, although we argued with him about this. (We were adolescents: At that age you argue about everything.) We thought it would be difficult to keep those secrets. There was a difficult period of give-and-take, but eventually we got him to tell us one of the rules. And this is the one I'll tell you.

What I'm going to tell you is the first piece of advice he gave. I heard it the first morning I ever spent in the hospital. It's a memory that smells of oranges. I like it when memories have a smell.

He asked us to sit up, looked at both of us, and said:

"Write this down. In this life you've got to know how to say no."

The guy from the Canary Islands and I looked at each other: We didn't understand a thing. How to say no? And anyway, why did we have to say no, when it's so great to say yes?

Next, just as he would do on the next six nights, he gave us a long explanation about why you have to say no. I wrote down the following:

- No to what you don't want.
- No to what you don't yet know that you don't want but at the moment you do want.
- No to obligations.
- No if you know you won't be able to fulfill what you're being asked to do.
- And most important: Say no to yourself!!!

I think that saying no to yourself must have been the most important one because he made us put down lots of exclamation marks after it. Next to the last exclamation mark there's even a stain made by a segment of orange (or that's what I think when I look at it). Sometimes what one wants is so intense that it becomes a reality.

The day after giving us the seventh piece of advice, he died. It was one of those deaths that mark you: He gave us seven rules to be happy and then he died. The guy from the Canary Islands and I were both aware of what he had left us. We decided to make a pact: We'd never lose the notes he'd made us take, and when we understood them we'd put them to use.

I forgot about these pieces of advice about being happy for years. This posthumous list contained, although I didn't yet know it, all that you need to know to be happy. I started to understand them little by little and eventually internalized them.

I can assure you that I've said no to lots of things in my life: no to things in the hospital, no to things out of the hospital. I've never felt that a no should be a yes. But it's clear that when you say no and you are sure about it, success is almost assured.

Sometimes I want to feel that I'm about to die so that I can tell people the other six rules. My friend from the Canary Islands was lucky like this: He died six years later and with a smile told me that he had passed the rules on to three other people. He was a great guy, who didn't speak all that much: He thought that words were overrated.

The list of nos:

1. You have to know how to say no.
2. Nos have to have to do with things that you want, that you don't want, that you know aren't anything to do with you, and that are also relevant to you.
3. Nos have to be accepted. Don't doubt yourself; if you say no, trust the no that you say.
4. Enjoy the nos as much as the yeses. Nos don't have to be negative; they can make you happy, they can build the same bridges as the yeses. Don't think that you are

denying anything, but rather that you are opening up the way to other yeses.

The last thing I wrote down in the notebook was "Don't fool yourself: a no will bring you lots of yeses." When I was fourteen I didn't understand anything, but now that I'm thirty-four I think I've got a meaning worked out. I want to make it as far as sixty to see what new meanings appear out of what he told me. Every year, the list of seven rules gathers more meanings, shows a different face to the world. This is the good thing about age: It changes everything. I think this is the greatest thing about getting older, about becoming an adult.

Every year I go back over those notes, getting more and more juice out of the seven rules to happiness. Enjoy the first one. One out of seven isn't bad.

8

What you hide the most reveals the most about you

Tell me a secret and I'll tell you why you're so special.
—Néstor,
the coolest orderly I ever met

We're all special. I know it sounds like a cliché, but we are. We never liked hearing the words *disabled* or *invalid* in the hospital. They're two words to get rid of; lack of physical function doesn't have anything to do with them.

Over the years I have worked with mentally handicapped people, and here's another phrase to get rid of. These are people who tend to be the most special of all and the ones I respect the most; they're sensitive, innocent, and simple. And I use these words in their most positive sense. They're special.

I'm missing a leg and a lung, although I've always thought that in fact I had an artificial leg and a single lung. Missing, possessing—it all depends on how you look at it. In my own way I am special. I like to think that I'm marked out in some way and that this makes me different.

But it's not just the lack of physical or mental elements that makes someone special. Like I said earlier, we're all special. All you have to do is validate what it is that makes you special.

There was an orderly in the hospital who said: "Tell me a secret and I'll tell you why you're so special." While we were in the recovery rooms he told us about special people and the secrets that we all have. He thought that secrets are necessary in life, that they are private treasures only available to each of us individually. Because no one knows them, there's no key to get to them, and they mark us internally because we never share them.

Above all he told us of the importance of sharing our secrets. He said it was like showing other people what makes us special, what makes us different, and that's always the most difficult thing to talk about.

While he explained these things to us I looked at him closely. I wanted to know what this dark-skinned man was thinking, with his round eyes and prominent eyebrows. I wanted to know why he was special, what the secrets were that made him different.

I never knew what they were, but he taught us something vital: The things that we had—false legs, scars, bruises, bald heads—these were things that made us different and made us feel special, which is why we should never hide them but show them with pride.

He achieved his aim: I've never been ashamed to show off the things I lack. And I've been able to make secrets, the things that are the most difficult for us to share, nothing more than a proof of our differences.

When I left the hospital I didn't forget these lessons. Whenever I've had a secret I've asked myself if having it is a good idea and I've decided when to reveal it, when to allow it to transform me into someone special. What you hide is what says the most about you.

The formula is . . .

1. Think about your most hidden secrets.
2. Allow them to mature and finally reveal them. Enjoy keeping them hidden, but enjoy it more when you show them.
3. When you do reveal them, secrets will make you special. Whatever they were, they used to be yours and now they belong to lots of people.

9

Put your lips together and blow

It's not just for your birthday. Blow and make a wish, blow and make a wish.
—the mother of my friend Antonio, one of the Eggheads, who left us at the age of thirteen

It's possible that while I was in the hospital they gave me a thousand injections, no kidding. I've got cysts, dry veins, hidden veins. I love it when a vein decides to sink down into the body's catacombs, far away from the skin, far away from the needles. How intelligent veins are.

I always breathed out when they gave me an injection, as much when I stopped feeling pain as when I felt it. Breathing out, like blowing out a candle, always makes things better. I like to think there's something magical in it.

I remember that Antonio's mother—Antonio was a funny little Egghead who always made me laugh—told us that we should blow out air and make a wish. She told us that people only do this when it's their birthday because they think that there's something powerful about the day itself, but they don't know that it's the blowing out that's the most important thing. I loved Antonio's mother; she always told us great stories full of examples. Among many other things, she told us about the power of blowing on things.

She told us about mothers who blew on their children's injuries when they fell off their bicycles, about grazes that were cured with nothing more than blowing and a little bit of hydrogen peroxide. Blowing on things as a superpower.

I believed this without question. Every time they gave me an injection I made a wish; I never forgot to do this. I blew out, made a wish, and noticed the injection. I smiled automatically. What luck it was to be able to make so many wishes. I felt privileged. Also, I should add, lots of them have been fulfilled.

And now in my normal life I haven't stopped blowing. I blow and make a wish two or three times a week, without any obvious cause, whenever I need to. As Antonio's mother said, all these wishes, all this blowing accumulates inside us and we have to let it out, we have to extract these desires.

So don't be frightened, and blow at least once a week, whenever you need to make a wish.

Sometimes I think that so many of my wishes have come true because of blowing so much in the hospital.

I think that, without knowing, the body has given us a weapon against bad luck; the problem is that the day-to-day nature of this superpower stops us from noticing it.

Remember:

1. Form your lips into an O.
2. Think of a wish and believe that perhaps it will come true. The wish has to be something that you really want; it can't be just anything.
3. And blow. Breathe out air, your own air. And remember, the bigger the wish, the bigger the amount of air you blow out. The ideal is for you to breathe out until there's nothing left inside. End up without any more air to blow out.

I'm sure that the people who live to be a hundred have blown out like this a lot. This exchange of air, breathing in and out, is what has given them such long lives.

Antonio died blowing out. I don't know what he was wishing for, but his mother told me that she was sure his wish had been granted. I believe so, too. Put your lips together and blow. Make another wish. . . .

10

Don't be afraid of being the person you have become

Albert, trust the person you used to be. Respect your past self.

—one of the cleverest doctors I had
(this was what he told me while he was
explaining what the surgery would be like)

My doctor always told me that he wanted the best for me, but sometimes what seemed the best ended up not being the best. It's difficult to know how a human body will react to a drug, or a therapy or an operation. But he asked me to trust him, and he emphasized this: "I've always believed," he said, "that if my 'past me' took this decision, it was because he believed in it. [Your 'past you' is you a few years, months, or days ago.] Respect your past you."

This was a great piece of advice. Maybe at that exact moment I didn't think of it in that way. I was about to have an operation and I really hoped that his "present him" wasn't going to make a mistake.

After I left the hospital I reflected on these words. It was a great discovery, not just for medical purposes but for everything. We tend to think that we make the wrong decisions; it's as if we think that we're cleverer now than we used to be, as if our past selves hadn't balanced all the pros and cons of the decisions we made.

Ever since that doctor told me about his past self, I've always believed in my past me. I even think he's cleverer than my future me. So when I sometimes make a wrong decision I don't get annoyed; I remember that I made the decision myself and that it was considered and thought through (one thing is true, I always try to think through and consider my decisions).

You mustn't be upset by the wrong decisions you make. You have to trust your past you. Of course your fifteen-year-old you could have made a mistake not taking that class, or your twenty-three-year-old you shouldn't have gone on that trip, or your twenty-seven-year-old you shouldn't have taken that job. But it was you who made those decisions and you must have dedicated some time to making them. Why do you think that you've now got the right to judge what he, your past you, decided to do? Accept who you are; don't be afraid of being the person that your decisions have made you into.

Bad decisions crystallize; bad decisions, after a while, turn into good decisions. Accept this and you will be happy in your life and, above all, happy with yourself.

My doctor made three or four mistakes. I never threw

these decisions in his face because I didn't think that his mistakes came from a lack of experience or professionalism. In order to make mistakes, one has to take risks; the result is the least important part of the process.

I am sure that if we got your eight-year-old you, your fifteen-year-old you, and your thirty-year-old you together in a room, they would have different ideas about almost everything and they would be able to justify every decision they'd made. I love trusting my past me; I love living with the results of the decisions he made.

I have a huge scar over where my liver is from surgery. The operation wasn't any use in the end because there was nothing wrong with my liver, but my doctor had thought I had cancer and that if I wasn't operated on then I would die. This scar makes me feel very proud, makes me feel a lot of different feelings whenever I see it. Everything that provokes a surge of emotions is positive, extremely positive.

So:

1. Analyze any decisions you've made that you think were mistakes.
2. Remember who made them. If it was you, remember the reasons you had. Don't believe that you are cleverer than your past you.
3. Respect your decisions and live with them.
4. Eighty percent of you is the consequence of decisions you've made. Love yourself for what you are; love yourself for what you have become.
5. Above all, acknowledge that you sometimes make mis-

takes. The 20 percent of you made out of mistakes is
something you have to acknowledge and accept.

Like that doctor told me: *Acknowledgment* is the key
word. You have to acknowledge yourself, acknowledge how
you became what you are, and acknowledge whose fault it is.

They taught us in the hospital to accept that we can make
mistakes. My doctor sometimes made mistakes and always
accepted the blame. The world would run more smoothly if
we all accepted that we make mistakes, that we have made
mistakes, that we're not perfect. Lots of people try to find
excuses for their mistakes, look for someone else to blame,
shift liability for deaths onto other people; they never know
the joy of accepting responsibility. There is joy in the knowledge that you have made a wrong decision and that you acknowledge it.

I would love to see more trials where people admit their
guilt, or drivers stopped for breaking the speed limit admit
that they were going too fast.

We have to acknowledge that we make mistakes in order
to see where the mistakes are and not make them anymore.
Maybe lots of people are afraid of the punishment that will
follow from this admission, but the punishment is the least
important bit; the only important thing is to give your brain
the correct information.

11

Find what you like looking at, then look at it

Wowwww!
—exclamation produced by the little Egghead Marc,
the youngest one (as a silver car parked
millimeters away from him)

There was a five-year-old kid who they brought into the hospital with cancer of the tibia. Sometimes he came with us to "the sun." "The sun" was a place that they'd set up next to the parking lot; it always caught the sun and there was a basketball hoop.

It wasn't easy to get permission to go to the sun. You had to behave very well. They normally let us be in the sun between five and seven. I loved going out of the hospital to go to the sun. It made me feel great, like going on a trip to New York: The contrast was huge. We stayed out for those two hours taking the sun; we got tanned.

Sometimes the little guy came with us. But he didn't lie

down to take the sun like the rest of us. He stayed standing up, staring at the parking cars. If people parked well, he went crazy; his eyes got as big as saucers; he smiled and laughed and clapped like mad. If they took a long time parking or had to flail around a lot, he went crazy the other way; he got angry and almost ended up kicking the car.

I don't know where this passion for cars came from, but as time went on we stopped tanning ourselves and just stared at him. He was worth watching. He was passionate, intelligent, observant; he was a mystery to us.

I think that he didn't look just at cars; he looked at movement, looked at time, turns, elegance. This is what made him crazy: shapes, the energy in the turns, the sweetness of a perfect piece of parking.

A few months later they detected that the cancer had metastasized in both his lungs. That day we went down to the sun together. He didn't have permission but we managed to smuggle him out with a false permission slip that another patient had left.

I knew that he liked looking at the cars. We spent almost two hours there in the sun, watching them park. When we were heading back to the hospital I asked him: "Why do you like looking at cars so much, Marc?" He looked at me and asked: "Why do you all like looking at the sun so much?" I said that it wasn't so much that we looked at the sun but that the sun gave us . . . it was nice . . . that . . . The truth is I didn't know why we looked at the sun.

Not to judge: That's the important lesson that kid taught me that day. He looked at cars and I looked at the sun. I kept quiet and he went crazy about what he saw. I'm sure that his

cars gave him as much as the sun gave me: color, health, happiness. I imagine that watching people park cars gives you
some sort of pleasure as well. The important thing isn't what
you look at, but what you get out of looking.

I got very angry that day, cried so much that night. . . . I
didn't want that kid to die in a couple of months. The way
that boy looked at things had to survive, had to get him as
far as running countries, leading men. There was something
in his passion that dazzled me. I don't know what became of
him. So I hope that wherever he is he's still looking at things
with the same passion.

I never judged anyone again. I just enjoy other people's
passions. I have friends who like looking at birds, looking at
walls, looking at the waveforms emitted by cellphones.

Find what you like looking at and look at it.

12

Start counting at six

Change your brain!
—idea given me by a neurologist in blue pajamas
just before they gave me a CAT scan

They took three CAT scans of my brain. You have to stay very still. I tried not to think about anything personal; I was scared that the machine would print it. I knew that the machines didn't print these things out, but I felt that everything was being recorded, so I didn't think about anything.

One summer, the summer of the World Cup when Gary Lineker was the star, I spent three hours waiting in the hospital and the only thing that I could think of was that I was missing one of the semifinals. I was sure that when they did the CAT scan they'd see Lineker and his goals and the whole stadium going wild.

There was a man there who looked at me. He was an older man with little eyes. He was wearing blue pajamas like me. We started to talk to each other: "They're taking ages. Is it for a CAT scan?" It's that sort of question that brings people together in waiting rooms.

We went to sit next to each other. Neither of us went to where the other one was but we both went to a third place. He told me he was a neurologist. The conversation we had was about the brain, the famous 10 percent of the brain that we use. This is something that has always bothered me; I want our successors to be able to use 30 or 40 percent. In the end we'll go down in history as the guys who used only 10 percent, the ones with the sticks and the rocks and the 10 percent, that's those guys, over there. We've come a long way, but for the people of the thirtieth century we'll be primitives.

This neurologist told me that in order to use more of the brain all we have to do is change our brain.

If you say the words *change* and *brain* to a fifteen-year-old boy, then you'll get his attention pronto. "How can you do it? I want to change my brain."

He spoke to me about numbers. It was a simple example. He showed me four objects: In this case it was four magazines. He asked me to count them. I said that there were four of them. He asked me: "Did you need to think?" I said no, that it was easy. I started to wonder if he really was a neurologist; he was more like a patient from Floor 8 (Psychiatry). He showed me five magazines and asked me to count them. Suddenly I realized that my brain had started to work. I was counting: I couldn't do it without counting. He smiled at me, and his eyes grew even narrower: "You're counting, right?" I looked at him in amazement.

He explained to me that when you get to five, our 10 percent of the brain starts to count. The way to exercise it is to try to make it start counting at six, and then at seven. In this way we force it to increase its capacity, so more neurons fire up when we use our brain. We change it a little bit at a time, so that it isn't so weak, so that we notice it start working.

I wanted more. He spoke to me about when you see nine people and have the sensation of a group. Up to eight, you don't think of them as a group, but when you hit nine your brain identifies them as a little crowd. Another way to change your brain: Make it start seeing a crowd when you hit fifteen, or even twenty.

I said it was like changing the factory settings of something. Was it possible? He told me that we were talking about a brain, that it didn't have factory settings and that all changes were possible.

They called me for the CAT scan. I knew that when I came out I wouldn't find him again. This happened a lot in the hospital: You'd go away for a minute and a person you'd made a connection with would have disappeared.

As I was leaving I shouted to him: "I'm going to use fifteen percent of my brain! Twenty percent!" He smiled at me. A moment before they shut the door to the room where they were going to test me I noticed sadness, a huge sadness flooding from him. I don't know what it was, but it made me tremble; this man radiated something.

They shut me into the CAT scanner and asked me not to move. I remember that this was the first day I started to change my brain. Every time it tells me something is definite I reject it and change what my brain thinks is the correct answer. I am in dialogue with my brain and have changed its factory settings.

Over time I have realized that this man was not sad but was instead very happy. My brain thought that his lost gaze, his stare, radiated sadness. That was the factory setting. But it was actually happiness; he was happy to hear a kid of fifteen shout out the phrase that he most believed in.

Does this discovery help in our daily life? It's really useful. You could put it this way: Don't obey your first thoughts blindly. Consider well what it is that you are thinking. Look for things; don't just be happy with your first thought.

It is possible to change your brain. I have trained myself to start counting at six; maybe it doesn't seem like much, but I'm very proud.

So, don't believe anything that comes straight from the factory. Think about it carefully and your life will improve.

13

The search for the south
and the north

*Dreams are the north for everyone; if they come true
then you've got to head south.*
—an intensive care nurse who stroked my hair
as I realized that I only had one lung

This is a piece of advice that speaks for itself.

I don't want to spend a lot of time on something that's so obvious.

Where did I hear it? In the intensive care unit. I'd just come out of the lung operation and I had lost lung capacity—one of my lungs was missing. What did they do with it? I've always asked myself that.

A nurse came up and looked at me. She stroked my hair. I liked it a lot. Through the mask I tried to thank her for her kindness, but I'm sure that my face was made stupid by the anesthetic and I must have said just the opposite.

She was talking to another nurse who was stroking the

big toe on the only foot I had left. I swear I'm not making it up. It was a bit sexy, but it was great to wake up to such kindness after losing a lung.

The younger girl said to the older one: "Dreams are the north for everyone; if they come true then you've got to head south."

That sentence fascinated me so much! I almost couldn't breathe. . . . Luckily I was on a respirator so I didn't have to worry about it.

They left, and I thought: How much north have I got left to travel? How much south will I conquer once my dreams have come true?

In my life outside the hospital I've put this into practice. Sometimes, if you're lucky enough for your dreams to come true, you'll see how you reach the north. I envisage the north of my life, and then I look for another dream and tell myself: "This must be in the south."

I know, I was sedated and two nurses were stroking me. Should I trust so much in a piece of advice obviously influenced by external circumstances? The answer is yes; in fact, maybe I should obey it all the more because it touched me so deeply.

North and south. Nothing more. Look for the north; look for the south. Don't stop traveling between them.

14

Listen to yourself when you're angry

My father didn't have a car but we went to the car
pound every Saturday to shout at the guard. It's fun.
—Jordi, an Egghead whose hair never fell out.
Strange kid.

Sometimes you've got to let it all out. It's a law of life. Shout three or four times into the air. Either that or you'll explode.

There was an Egghead in the hospital who told us that he sometimes went with his father to the car pound; his father would shout at the duty officer there. He'd say that they should be ashamed of themselves, that they wanted to make him pay 120 euros; he got angry and shouted to the heavens. After ten minutes or so they'd head off. The police had never taken his dad's car; it was just that the dad had found a place where he could go to let off steam. The wrong place? Well, of course the poor duty officer didn't deserve that kind of explosion of anger directed at him. Sometimes I think about those police officers, or the people who deal with lost luggage at an airport. Where do *they* go to let off steam? How can they want to go to work each morning?

I think that the father of Jordi the Egghead (an Egghead with hair—weird, weird) went to the wrong place: There must be easier ways to blow off some steam. In the hospital we sometimes shouted at a tape recorder. It was the idea of one of the cancer residents who came to see us every Saturday.

He was young and wanted to change the world. Now he's the head of the department and the armor plating that most doctors end up wearing has made him forget all that. But I'm here to remind him about it. It's good when people remind you of the worthwhile things you've done.

The resident brought a tape recorder and we took turns letting it rip. We said everything that really upset us. There were some of us who found a lot to shout about. For instance, it's terrible when you think they're going to give you a pass for the weekend and they end up not giving it to you. We shouted; we got rid of everything that was annoying us and getting us down. Other people said nothing; they just looked at you.

Then the resident made us listen to the recording. It was always a fascinating moment: to hear yourself shouting, to hear yourself angry, sounding like a madman, paranoid. Suddenly, everything that had seemed to make sense, that you would have defended a second ago, seemed baseless. It was as if your anger dissipated with the echo of your rage.

The echo of rage has this power: the power to minimize

your anger, the power to show you how ridiculous it is to shout and throw your toys out of the stroller.

Who better than you to put up with all your shouting? Try it, you'll feel better; and little by little you'll stop shouting, stop getting annoyed, and, above all, you won't shout at other people. You'll see how ridiculous you are when you get like that.

15

Positive wanking

You are who you really are after a wank.
—a physiotherapist who didn't manage to
give me bigger quadriceps but who
was a funny guy nonetheless

I'm very much in favor of wanking. A few years ago I wrote a play called *Wank Club*. My passion for wanking comes from the bad press that it gets. People always talk about wanking a bit disrespectfully, as a joke, as if it were something from the second division.

I'm extremely interested in wanking, especially what people hide behind it. Sometimes it's unrecognized passion, sometimes it's excessive love, sometimes it's sex, sometimes shame, sometimes hidden desires. Wanking always tells you more about a person than all the personal details you ask them.

"You are who you really are after a wank." A physiotherapist told me this. He explained that after having a wank all that is left is what is really you. In those two or three minutes after masturbating the essence of who you really are appears.

He also said: "A wank is like an externalized suicide. It's like killing yourself from the outside." He was a very tall man, nearly seven feet tall, and he spoke about wanking like other people talk about soccer or the movies. He spoke about it with such passion that it was impossible not to listen to him. I really like discovering what someone's passion is; passion is what interests me the most.

It must have been him who first made me interested in wanking, and this interest has never faded. I think that you wank when you feel good and also when you feel terrible. It's something invariable in life, a form of channeling energy.

The physiotherapist was a fan of "positive wanks," which, according to him, are wanks that make you think of another person and bring him or her luck. If you dedicate your wank to someone, your luck passes to them.

This way of focusing your wanks has always seemed to me poetic. So many positive wanks in my life! You feel powerful, as if you have a gift.

So go ahead, don't be afraid. Just make yourself think about only one person. And let magic do the rest.

16

The difficult thing isn't accepting how you are, but how everyone else is

Some people vomit and some people don't vomit.
—great sentence delivered by a nurse
(that day I was vomiting)

Well, this discovery is in fact two discoveries, two in one.

1. Accept who you are. It's not easy, I know. Saint Augustine said: "Know yourself, accept yourself, better yourself." I think he was extremely optimistic to think you could do all three things. I've always been happy with knowing myself. It's not easy to know yourself, to know what your desires are, what things you like, what things you don't enjoy.

   But it is possible. Give it time, search, search again, keep searching, and eventually you'll have a picture-perfect portrait of who you are.

2. Once you know yourself, if you manage to develop

some affection for yourself, the hard bit comes next. The second part of the discovery: Know everyone else and accept them for who they are.

I know this might seem a little bit like a religious commandment, but in fact I simply mean that you should have the same patience with other people as you have been able to have with yourself. Accept what they are, accept what they are not: It's the first step toward accepting what you are like, what you are not like.

And this is where the rest of the chapter heading comes from. The most difficult thing isn't accepting what you're like, but what all the other people are like. This is the aim. Sometimes, when we know a few people, we might think we have reached our goal. But the goal's a long way away, still very distant. Every day we will meet more and more people and we will have to dedicate all our efforts to understanding them.

This discovery, which seems so complicated, came from a nurse. There was a guy who managed not to vomit when he had chemotherapy, and from that day on he got annoyed when there were other people around him who were vomiting. He didn't try to understand and get to know other people; he'd attained his objective and as far as he was concerned the rest of humanity was just trailing in his wake. The nurse told him that some people vomit and others don't vomit. And that's where it all started.

She managed to get the guy who didn't vomit to tell us some of his tricks; one of them was to drink Coca-Cola, which he claimed was a great antivomitory measure.

It was amazing to see him give advice. Sometimes it's not so important to follow a path as to leave the path we've been following, choose another one, and realize that there's more than one way to get where we're going. Don't judge; try not to be absolute. Every path can be good; it just has to be clearly the product of a particular decision.

17

The power of contrasts

We're not going to die of cancer; we're going to die of boredom!
—one of our favorite chants

On the fourth floor of the hospital where I was always sent as an inpatient, we dreamed of things we didn't have.

A long time after that I've given talks in hospitals, and lots of patients have said the same thing: There isn't enough stuff in the hospital, there's no fun.

We used to say in the hospital that we weren't going to die of cancer but rather of boredom. It's because everyone thinks that when you're in a hospital your life has to stand still, that you shouldn't have any fun. And the truth is completely the opposite. Your normal life stands still and so you need many more activities to fight against all this not living.

I remember when people were saying that the late-night talk show *The Martian Chronicles* was trash. I think that all those critics must never have been in a hospital where they were showing it. Thousands of sick people laughed with that program, enjoyed it. It gave them strength; it gave them life. It made them participants in a world that had stepped away from them for a moment.

It's always seemed to me that not much imagination goes into designing hospitals. When I started treatment, the chemotherapy rooms didn't have any sort of entertainment at all. Later there was a little television set looking over the room, but you had to be eagle-eyed to see it.

But where were the chessboards, the board games, the cards, the fifty-inch plasma TVs, the consoles, the Wi-Fi connection? Yes, yes, no joke, there should be all these things in a hospital. Connecting people to the world is vital in helping them fight illness properly.

Sometimes people don't realize how much life force patients have. I've always recommended that patients should give talks themselves. They've had experiences that would leave you astounded. In the hospital, I'm sure that if there was a talk given by someone from outside, then you'd go, so just imagine that it's a proper talk, but it's your roommate in his blue pajamas right next to you giving it.

When you're sick your second life appears. A life that you can't stop living, because however ill you are you've got to carry on being alive. I've had my life outside and my life inside. Now I'm living my life outside, but maybe my life inside will start again someday. Both lives have aspects in common but are very different in other ways. To carry on living is the important thing. Childhood, adolescence, adulthood: They all have to be lived through, even if you are ill.

But you need the track to be able to run, you need the stage to be able to act. Sometimes hospitals lack contrast, and the most important thing about life is putting contrasting things together. I've always thought that when you put two opposing things together, something magical happens. This is why lots of relationships are founded on the complete lack of common ground between the two members of the couple.

We should put more contrasting things together. These are a few that I hope will soon happen. The list's not in any order; it's a list that comes from years spent in a hospital and years spent outside one:

1. Olympic-sized swimming pools in hospitals. So many patients would get so much out of swimming! You can dive under the water and feel like a fish.
2. Bowling alleys in airports. It's important to be able to let off steam. You'd feel great relaxing with a few lanes. Sports and airports, any sport would be good in an airport. (They are starting to build gyms in airports. They must be doing a whole lot of good.)
3. Hairdressers in cinemas. You could get a good haircut before going to see a movie. *I'm going to get a haircut and catch a film.* It would be great if there were someone who recommended a new style to you or a shave or just a massage and a bit of depilation. *What film are you going to see? Well, I recommend you have this particular style.*
4. Books in woods. Little libraries in the middle of forests. Books originally come from forests; we should

leave some there. Make some cupboards and put them there. It would be great if you could climb a mountain and find the perfect book to read when you got to the top.

5. Bars in banks. Little bars while you wait to take money out or see if they're going to give you a loan. Why do banks have to be so serious; why can't there be a bar so that you can meet other clients, know what they're interested in, what they hope to get out of their life or their investments? I'm sure loads of people would go in the morning and say happily: "I'm just off to the bank; I'll be back in ten minutes." Have a nice cup of coffee or a quick snack before deciding what to do with your savings. On one side you order a little plate of squid and on the other two hundred thousand euros: See which one you get first.

18

Hibernate for twenty minutes

Don't move. Breathe, don't breathe.
—phrase most likely to be heard
in any X-ray room

There are phrases in the hospital that you hear until you're fed up with them; they end up forming part of you. It's as if they were suddenly in fashion. It's like when there's a phrase that gets famous on a TV program and then people don't stop repeating it. In the hospital world it's the same sort of thing; this is one of those phrases.

"Don't move. Breathe, don't breathe" is what you hear most often when they give you an X-ray or a CAT scan. They above all need you not to move; you have to stay very still so that everything shows up in the right place. This period of immobility lasts between fifteen minutes and an hour and fifteen minutes. You have to be very patient to get much out of these moments; you have to take them as moments of inner peace.

Of course, to enjoy having cancer you have to enjoy dead time, which is the basis for everything when you've got this illness. It's the hardest thing: to not do anything, to stay still even though inside you really want to walk away, to fly, to play, to work.

This is what you have to control, and this is also what it's most difficult to accept. You're alone in the room, because no one else wants to irradiate themselves. What about me? Do I want to irradiate myself? I always asked myself that when the others left the room.

But it's not just about being still, it's also about keeping quiet.

And as if that weren't enough, you have to control not only your silence but also your breathing. Lots of silence, lots of stillness, and lots of controlled breathing.

Without knowing it, every time they gave me an X-ray I came into contact with my inner self. It was like looking for something and finding it: self-examination, a strange yoga that made me feel better. I came out of the X-ray room improved.

And so, after I was cured, I carried on using this method. Every month I try to make an appointment to give myself an X-ray. I don't actually have an X-ray machine at home, but they're not necessary for you to examine yourself from the inside.

1. I lie down on my bed. I shut all the doors, turn off my cellphone, and stay still, very still.

2. I repeat in my mind the number one phrase from the hit parade: "Don't move. Breathe, don't breathe."

3. I do this for twenty minutes. I forbid myself from doing anything that isn't thinking about not moving or rationing the air that I breathe.

4. And, magically, when you finish this period of not doing anything, you can solve problems that had become rusted shut, find feelings that you had thought lost forever, and believe (of course, you have to check it later) that you have the solution for everything.

It might seem like meditation, but really it's just being still. Everything in this world would be a great deal better if we just stayed still for a while, stayed very still. Twenty-minute hibernations.

19

Look for your hospital roommates outside of the hospital

You're my brother, my little brother from the hospital!
—my hospital brother Big Antonio, a singer

I've been lucky enough to have great roommates. In another chapter I'll speak about some of them. They're like brothers you have for hours, or days or months. They really are like brothers, potential "yellows."

I love the feeling of coming into a room dressed in your street clothes, finding someone unknown (wearing pajamas and with his closest family members around his bed), and knowing that in a few days you'll be intimate friends.

Every time you get to a hospital they give you the bed closest to the window. It's like an unwritten rule, but they know that you'll need to go to the window and look at the world you're leaving behind for a bit. Another unwritten rule is that the patient doesn't have to get into pajamas on the

first day. The new arrival has twenty-four hours to acclima-
tize.

It's a struggle to take off your day clothes and go to bed at
noon when you feel well. Normally, after putting on the hospital pajamas, it takes you almost another twenty-four hours
to get into bed.

These first forty-eight hours are when your roommate
starts helping you. Sometimes with words, sometimes only
with gestures. Sometimes, simply and straightforwardly, by
explaining what he's got, what he felt when he arrived, and
what he's been feeling in the hospital. Experience is the basis
of communication; to see yourself reflected in someone else
means you're halfway to winning the battle.

My best roommate was called Antonio and he was from
Mataró. He had a huge hole in the sole of one foot, almost
big enough to hide a Ping-Pong ball. But he was all energy, all
nerves. He had more energy than almost everyone I've met
since.

He was nineteen and I was fourteen. He made me laugh a
lot. He let me spend almost four days without getting into
pajamas and protected me from the doctors and the nurses;
he said he liked seeing me dressed, that it made him feel as if
he had a visitor.

He had a little piano that he used to play songs, and little
by little, using music, he started to help me. He would play
and I would sing. We wrote great songs. Our most successful
one was "Give Me a Weekend Off" and our next-biggest hit
was "Write Me a Ticket for the Sun."

He was an amazing person who, without knowing it, was

fading a little every day. Every day there were fewer doctors who came to visit him and more people who came from outside. This is the clearest sign that you're dying: when friends start to visit you at all times and the doctors ration their visits because they haven't got much to tell you.

He spoke to me about women and love. It was his favorite topic: how to find the perfect woman, how to find the love of your life. When he had only two days left he was still looking for it, still philosophizing about it. I think it was love that made him so special; the search was reflected on his face.

He died. I didn't see him die. We never saw them die: They almost always went home to die. We knew that when they left they would die, but we said goodbye to them when they were still alive; that was always very good.

He left me his piano; he said that one day it would be worth millions. I still have it; I still play it. There's no doubt he also left me some of his energy. I didn't share it with him, I asked for it all; I asked for it and he gave it to me. It's inside me still and I'm sure that it's 90 percent of all the passion I have.

I had twenty roommates. Nineteen were great; one was horrible. (He snored, he didn't talk much, and when he did he was dull; he just kept on repeating: "I am a human being.") The other nineteen have influenced me. It's a positive statistic.

I'm still looking for roommates. I think it's what I look for most of all. You can find roommates in real life; you just need to know that you won't find them in a hospital but somewhere else: in an elevator, at work, in a shop.

Because yellows (and we will talk about them in detail at the proper time) are the foundations of the world.

The important thing to do is to look for them, to look for these roommates.

1. Find a stranger. Someone who powerfully attracts your attention.
2. Talk to them. Simply talk. Say what comes into your mind. Find a way to approach him or her, gently, very gently.
3. Give them forty-eight hours. People always need forty-eight hours to lower their defenses, to trust you, to get into their pajamas, to accept someone.
4. Enjoy your roommate.

But this is just a start. If you find roommates outside the hospital, then you can find everyone else: the orderlies, the doctors, the nurses, the yellows.

I don't mean to say that you need to find doctors outside the hospital and make friends with them; I mean that there are people who can have the same effect on you as the doctor has on your body and your illness.

1. For me, finding doctors means finding people who can cure you or listen to you. They're necessary; they're part of the yellow network, the network of friends. But you have to be able to divide them, set them to one side, so that you know that you can approach these yellow doctor friends when you are "unwell."

2. Nurses are people who can go with you anywhere, give you moral support, or share with you all the thousands of problems you have. They're the kind of people you end up thanking for something they've done thousands and thousands of times, because going somewhere boring with you on a sunny summer day when they could be on the beach is something that has no price.

3. Orderlies are individuals, lucky encounters, altruistic people who give you a hand at different moments of your life. It could be on the highway when your car breaks down, or it could be when they lend you money after a robbery. Lots of people call them charitable souls. I call them orderlies.

We will talk about the yellows at length in a bit. Patience, patience. Let's just build the hospital for the moment, the environment.

20

Do you want to share an REM with me?

Nighttime gives you the strength to change the rhythm of your life. All you need to know is what you want to change and that the dawn will not come soon.
—Christian, somebody's brother
(I've forgotten whose)

Nights are the yellowest part of the day. I like nights because almost everything is made real.

Nights in the hospital were great. They were calm. For years the Eggheads escaped at night: We took our wheelchairs and went looking for adventure, running all over those six vast floors.

We didn't have wheels, we couldn't go to the disco, but we had wheelchairs and so many places to visit and play. Every day one of us would choose a place to go, where to spend the night. My favorite was going to see the "other" Eggheads: the newborn babies. We'd go, we'd whisper sweet nothings to them, we'd make them laugh, and they'd look at us and make their noises. It was a strange feeling: They had their whole lives ahead of them; ours were within touching distance of their end.

I've always believed in the power of the night; I'm sure that the night makes your wishes come true. There were so many nights in the hospital when I felt capable of overcoming my fears and changing the rhythm of my life, although this effort has only one obstacle in its way: You have to get past your dreams, avoid the cold light of day. This is where successful people live, people who turn their dreams into reality: They can overcome the dawn. This is what Christian always used to say. He was someone's brother but I can't remember whose. Sometimes the visitor is more important than the person visited.

I've always tried to have my best ideas born during the night: at three or four in the morning. This time of night is the right time to draw up plans. It's as if when you are almost ready to fall asleep your whole self is in agreement with what you are thinking, and this encourages you and gives you energy.

Being tired makes us sweeter. So many good ideas don't seem so good the next morning; so often the things we decide in the night fail to take place. I think that tiredness makes us less animal and more human, but I'm not sure if that's a good thing or not.

While I was in the hospital I made all my important decisions in these watches of the night, before falling asleep. I loved waking up at that time, when the whole hospital would be asleep, including the nurses; it was as if the whole place belonged to me. I planned my life, worked on my dreams, and aspired to do everything.

When I left the hospital I went back to doing this. I trusted a great deal in the middle of the night. Also, I'm sure that when someone invents a drug that stops you from needing to sleep, the middle of the night will be the time for a new meal: the REM.

The REM will be even more important than lunch or tea. You'll have REMs with people who are special, people who, like you, believe in this time of the day. When the moment comes I hope I'll be ready.

21

The power of the first time

"Moments" are our greatest treasure. They are what we are.
—a teacher who gave us lessons and spoke more about moments than math, because he thought that we'd forget about the math but the moments remain

He always started by saying, "There's nothing like a good moment. A moment is a piece of life we've all lived through."

I'm a big fan of moments, I'd say even more of a fan than that teacher (sometimes the pupil can be better than the master), because there was a time when I lost them. Moments occur most in childhood and adolescence. But everybody's life is full of moments.

There was a time while I was in the hospital when I stopped having moments; well, maybe that's not entirely true, but I exchanged them for other types of moment. Hospital moments, which I share with other people who've lived in hospitals.

"Moments" can be defined as things that one day you do for the first time and which mark you, because they stay with you.

For example, here's a triple moment connected to transport:

1. There's the first day that you and a friend left school together. The first time that you went out of school at the same time, talking about stuff. We've all experienced this moment: walking along with someone and then separating at some given point. It's a way of feeling adult. It's magic, a moment from when you were seven or eight years old.

2. Years later, approaching sixteen, you have another moment connected with going home. You don't walk home; you want to catch your first taxi. You go with a friend, you look for a taxi, you don't find one, you curse the ones that don't stop. It's another moment of maturity, of feeling yourself growing older.

3. And finally a day when you're about nineteen and you've got a car and you take a friend (maybe the same friend from the two previous moments) back to his house. And you sit with this friend talking in the car until the small hours. Another moment.

I think that there's nothing in life that I like more than looking for moments. After discovering them, after that teacher showed us what they were, I started to collect them. In the hospital, the moments I already had helped me to keep going. They happen at such a young age that they form the essence of your life. Every year I remember two or three moments and I feel good; I feel happy at this reencounter.

People sometimes forget that we are the fruit of what we live through in our childhood and our adolescence; we are the product of many moments. And sometimes we close the door to them when we should have it always open.

For a few years my moments were slightly strange: the first time my leg was amputated, the first time I lost a lung. But they were moments nonetheless.

And even when you are an adult, you live through a lot of moments, but what happens is that you stop noticing. I think that to truly know yourself you need to go back to your moments, analyze them, and accept them for what they are.

My life is made up of moments and odors, and they are what make me what I am.

22

A way never to get angry

Look for your point of no return.
—a radiologist with small ears and
huge eyebrows who hypnotized us with
his tone of voice and his stories

I think that there's nothing I hate more than getting angry: shouting, cursing, not being able to control myself.

Sometimes in the hospital we cursed our fate; sometimes we got angry about it. A doctor (a radiologist who sometimes told us jokes when he was on duty) taught us how to control our moments of anger, to be capable of knowing our limits.

He spoke to us about the "point of no return." Once you've passed this point, you can't avoid getting angry. It exists, it's tangible, it's physical; we can feel it and therefore we can control it.

Our radiologist friend made us take a piece of paper and

write down what it was we noticed before reaching this point, the levels of annoyance. What are they like? What do you notice when you feel that you can't control your fury?

It was a list of three or four points a bit like this:

1. I notice that I'm annoyed by what the other person is saying.
2. I start to notice that my anger is getting stronger.
3. I've started to raise my voice; I notice that my anger is getting control of me. I start to lose control.
4. I reach the point of no return.

If there are three stages before you get to this point, then you will see, just before you reach it, just before you lose control and get angry, that the possibility of stopping exists. Maybe you'll notice that just before the point of no return you move your hands a lot, or your voice shakes or you swear a lot. These are the effects you have to control.

How? First of all by asking your partner, or your friend or one of your yellows, to use a key word when they see one of these symptoms. They should say "pistachio" or "United States." Whatever it takes to make you realize that you are approaching the point. To begin with you don't notice your points of no return; they go by so quickly that the line between one state and the next is almost invisible.

When they've said the key word a few times you'll find that you start to become capable of hearing it. This is when you have to turn off your anger, take a step back, because if you don't reach that point then you'll be able to control yourself. Everything can be sorted out if you don't get to that point.

In the hospital I started to practice this; my key word was *tumor*. I've always liked giving a more positive spin to this word. Little by little I stopped getting annoyed. It worked, and I was overjoyed.

As you get older your point of no return changes position. As the years go by and we get more experienced we get angry less often and our point of no return is further away. So it is important to look for it: Every year you need to search for it, find it, and not go past it.

It's good to get angry every now and then, but it's not good to reach the point of no return.

23

The best way to know
if you love someone

Shut your eyes.
—Ignacio, a special one among
the special ones

This has to be one of the pieces of advice that fascinate me the most. On the third floor of the hospital there were special people, people unfairly known as the mentally handicapped. (I strongly believe that this phrase should be struck from the dictionary.)

I think that they're special people because they make you feel truly special. They are extremely innocent people who make everything simple and easy.

Perhaps what I found most exciting about them was seeing how they solved their problems, especially how they found out whether they loved someone. I've always thought that the great problems in our society come from the fact that people don't know whether they love the person they're with. This gives us a lot of headaches, lots of worries. Do I love the person I'm with or don't I? Are they the right person? Is there another person whom I like more? What should I do?

What you should do with such problems is what the special people do, what they taught me to do. It's nothing spectacular; it's not a great trick or something so surprising that it leaves your mouth hanging open.

Lots of times when we had problems we went to see the special people. There would always be a huge number of details that had nothing to do with the decision we had to make, and they knew how to detect these. They knew how to filter the details that were necessary for making the correct decision.

They always advised us to shut our eyes. For them, shutting the eyes was almost magical. You shut your eyes and it is as if you've managed to get rid of all the unimportant details. Closing your eyes eliminates one of your senses, the sense that distracts you most, that brings in the most information.

We shut our eyes a lot in the hospital. Now I do it more than ever: how much I've discovered, how many decisions I've made with my eyes shut! And the most incredible thing is that you see everything so clearly.

Twenty-three Discoveries That Connect Two Ages: From Fourteen to Twenty-four

These are the twenty-three discoveries and I hope that as you read each one you'll make more discoveries.

I hope that they give you the basis for this yellow world, the foundation for a different world.

I used them while I was getting cured, I set them running and they helped link two ages. You can use them to link two ages, too, or two moments or two sensations, or else just to live a single instant, the actual moment.

I remember that when I discovered them or started to put them into practice I was twenty-four. Just as I said at the beginning of the book, I was completely cured and couldn't believe it. A couple of days had gone by and I was completely disoriented: I knew who I was but not who I had been.

So I decided to bury myself in my childhood, in that fourteen-year-old pre-cancer kid, and to start to link the two ages: fourteen and twenty-four.

It was something magical, incredible. I returned to those memories, found what I had liked or desired, and it was as if I were transplanting them into a man of twenty-four. I spent a wonderful year building bridges, having a conversation between the two people who lived in this body. It was without doubt the most incredible year of my life: I listened to myself, understood myself, developed respect for myself. During this year I learned the lessons of cancer and applied them to my life. One of the two guys, the one who was twenty-four, had the weapons to fight cancer, and the fourteen-year-old had the innocence to keep on living as if he had never known cancer. What could be better than using both strengths together, both energies?

Of course, without cancer, the fourteen-year-old would have become someone different, and the twenty-four-year-old, who knew this, only wanted that younger kid to feel accepted, loved.

I liked it when they agreed on something, when they saw that there weren't so many things that separated them in reality. In fact, maybe they wanted the same thing but expressed it in different ways.

I also liked it when they argued; that was when I grew up, when I realized that I didn't now have the same objectives. And this was good, because somehow two people shared two interests, two aims. Debate is necessary to survive.

At the end of that year I made a pact with the fourteen-year-old: He would always have a vote, I would always listen to his opinion. Because that fourteen-year-old couldn't be what he'd wanted to be, I'd let him be with me always. And he's never abandoned me; I get older and bigger, but the fourteen-year-old kid is still inside me, advising me and giving me his opinion.

Without knowing it, many people forget their fourteen-year-old kid, but I think that the important thing is to go back, dive in, and build bridges back to that moment. It's like swimming along the bottom of a swimming pool, going through a little tunnel and ending up in a littler swimming pool; that's where the fourteen-year-olds are. Speak to them, exchange things with them, and rescue what you can for the larger pool.

The fourteen-year-old kids make us complicated, various. It's a difficult period, one in which we make our most important decisions, the decisions that mark our characters. The problem is that sometimes we forget; sometimes we think that we were mistaken and try to build ourselves from the beginning again.

I think it's good to build yourself up on the basis of what you already are: go back to the foundations, go back to the fourteen-year-old. The basis of what you are is certainly there. The basis of what you want to be. Now that I think about it, this could be another discovery, number twenty-four. But I'll leave it here.

Just trust in the twenty-three discoveries. Trust in them and they'll come true. And now let's go to the yellows. . . . The time has come!

Living . . .

The Yellows

Do you think it's right that an engineer should write poetry?
Culture is an ornament; business is business.
If you stay with that girl you're not welcome in our house.
That's living.

—Gabriel Celaya

The Yellows

We've reached one of the chapters that I think is the most important and that makes me the most excited to write. I'm very keen on talking about the yellows.

You have to know that it's 1:41 A.M. on an August night (when I revise the chapter it's 11:08 on an October morning). I've always believed that positioning the moment of writing, the day (it's early Thursday morning), gives everything a far greater reality. (The revision takes place midmorning on a Tuesday.) It's a dimension that you don't normally get when you read a book. When did he write this? Where was he? What was the weather like?

A few months ago I was lucky enough to interview Bruce Broughton, the composer of famous soundtracks for movies like *Young Sherlock Holmes* and *Silverado*. We spoke about the possible variables that can influence the creative process: your partner? The place? The temperature? He thought that above all creativity has to do with the way you receive what you see and how you transform it. Your own speed of transformation. It was really a great luxury to listen to someone who was so overflowing with creativity, although he acknowledged that his own speed of creation changed depending on whether he was alone or not, how hot it was, and how much he could concentrate.

But let's not get off the main topic: the yellows. As well as being a chapter of the book, they also give the book its original title. It's the great treasure that I gained from cancer. You can always learn something that takes you three steps or three miles further than the rest; there will always be an Induráin, a Borg;* there's always someone or something that stands out. And if you know, as I think you do, that I like lists, there has to be a well-ordered way of explaining why some things stand out.

This will be a long chapter, and because I don't want to get lost I'll try not to get sidetracked. Especially since if there's one thing I want you to take from reading this book, it's the idea of the yellows.

I hope that within a few months people will be looking for yellows, will use this term to describe them, will adopt it fully. There are words and phrases that appear and become popular, sometimes because of bad things (*tsunami*), sometimes because of good things (*Internet*), sometimes just because of the way fashions change (*metrosexual*). It's not that I particularly want to invent a new term, but I think it's necessary to have a word that defines this concept. Concepts

* Miguel Induráin ("Big Mig"): Spanish cyclist who won five consecutive Tours de France, 1991–95; Björn Borg: Swedish tennis player, winner of eleven Grand Slam singles titles between 1974 and 1981.

need words to define them, like people need names. There was a man in the hospital who always said: "They give you a name as soon as you're born; you can't not have a name!" I always looked at him and smiled—I didn't understand what he wanted to say. This happened to me a lot in the hospital; I was fifteen or sixteen and the other patients were pushing sixty or seventy. They spoke to me as if I were an adult, they gave me adult advice, they looked at me like an adult. And I wrote down everything I didn't understand but that I felt I might understand years later.

I love it when the brain decides to take in a concept, a language, a feeling. I think that the brain's on a time lock; you have to push lots of buttons and enter lots of different codes for it to open and accept what it at first rejected. All you need to do is find the password. The same way I hope to find what the yellows explain.

I met lots of yellows in the hospital, although I didn't know what they were back then. I thought that they were friends, twin souls, people who helped me, guardian angels. I didn't understand how a stranger who had played no part in your life until two minutes ago could suddenly become a part of you, understand you more than anyone else on this earth, and help you to feel completely identified with and understood. What I've just written could, plausibly, serve as an initial definition of a yellow.

This usually happened with my roommates. They quickly became my yellows. I don't know how long I spent talking with my roommates at ridiculous hours of the night. They were like detachable brothers. That's just it. I even called them that back then: hospital brothers, brothers with an expiration date. The intensity of our relationships was the sort that exists between brothers, and our friendships were very close.

But as the years went by I realized that the words *brother, friend, close acquaintance* weren't enough.

I remember a day in the hospital when two or three of us Eggheads were talking about our roommates. Someone defined them as angels; someone else said they were friends. Another guy and I said: "They're yellows." It came out at the same time. I don't know why we said yellows, but we felt strongly that this was the word that defined them. I'm a firm believer in chance and luck, and I think that chance is much stronger than luck. And I don't know if it was luck or chance, but I think that the only word that can truly define this concept is *yellow*.

I've never understood why the concept of friendship hasn't evolved. Sometimes I read books about the Middle Ages or the Renaissance, or about the beginning of this century, and they always talk about friendship in the same way: A friend is always a friend. Friends are friends and the relationship between friends is fairly similar at all times. On the other hand, the concepts of the couple or of the family have changed. The way in which we relate to a partner or a close family member nowadays has nothing to do with the way in which we related to them in the Middle Ages: Roles, customs, everything has evolved.

I think that this is one of the bad things about our society. The concept of friendship, the role of the friend: These need to change for the technological age we live in. I think that it's impossible to maintain contact now with friends in the same way you could in past decades. Everybody loses friends every year, and the excuses are very varied: We live in different countries; I got a new job; I don't have time to meet up; we only message each other from time to time; we were only friends in school or college.

Losing a friend is always connected with stopping seeing them. Friends are defined above all as people one sees, people you see a lot of in your life. Can you be friends with someone you never see, someone you never meet up with? In theory it's impossible. In theory.

For example, I always met my Egghead friends only in the hospital: It was a golden rule. We helped each other, we looked after each other, but when we left the hospital we had a pact not to see each other again. It's not that we forgot each other—quite the opposite, we kept each other inside ourselves—but we didn't need to keep on seeing each other. There were other things that tied us together.

It took me a long time to realize it, but these were the foundations of the yellows. One fine day I saw it clearly. There are friends who give you friendship; there are love affairs that give you passion, sex, or love; and, finally, there are yellows.

Perhaps you'll ask me if what I'm trying to say is that the yellows are substitutes for friends. The answer is no. Friends, traditional friends, still exist; we all have them. But there's a new rung on the ladder, a new concept: the yellows.

Everybody has yellows, but the problem is that until now there hasn't been a word to define them. I'm sure that yellows have always existed, but have just been lumped in with friends. Or sometimes a yellow turned into a lover. A yellow is in between a lover and a friend, and that's why things so often get confused.

Before I carry on, I'll give a definition of yellows. A definition of what I've explained up till now.

Yellow: A person who is special in your life. Yellows are found among your friends and lovers. It's not necessary to see them regularly or keep in touch with them.

According to this definition, how is it possible to distinguish between a friend and a yellow? Is there any way of knowing who is a friend and who is a yellow? In fact there is. You need a bit of practice and you need to know yourself quite well. Yellows are a reflection of you; they have some of the things you lack, and knowing them causes a qualitative leap forward in your life.

I'm going to tell you a little more about the yellows. Imagine that you are in an airport, in an airport in a foreign city. There's a delay, two or three hours. You're alone in this city and suddenly you start speaking to someone (a boy or a girl). To begin with it might just seem like a trivial conversation, but little by little you notice there's something between you; I'm not talking about love or sex, I'm talking about the feeling that you've met someone (a stranger) to whom you can tell the most intimate things and who understands you and advises you in a different and special way.

The plane's got to take off, so you've got to separate (in the best-case scenario you'll swap email addresses or cellphone numbers) and stop seeing each other. Maybe you'll write; maybe you'll send a message; maybe you'll never see each other again.

Traditionally, you couldn't consider such a person a friend—developing a friendship takes time, years. But maybe this person has given you more than a friend of six or seven years has; you've exchanged confidences and intense emotions. Also, one of the characteristics of a friendship is that seeing each other, regularly or at least assiduously, is important. And here you are meeting a stranger who affects you and makes you feel better, though you'll probably never see him again.

Normally such a situation causes sadness, a feeling of loss rather than gain, a feeling that you've found something and know that you have lost it. But really what you've done is gain a yellow. One of the twenty-three yellows you will have in your life.

So, what? A yellow is a stranger who understands me? Not exactly. A yellow can be someone you know, a yellow can be a friend who one day steps up the ladder to the level of yellow. It doesn't have to be a stranger. All it has to be is someone special who makes you feel special.

The most important thing is that a yellow doesn't need telephone calls, doesn't need to be looked after for years, doesn't need to be seen often (just once is enough for someone to become a yellow). So maybe there are lots of those people you don't see very often, who you don't think are your friends anymore because you don't have time to see them; maybe lots of them are your yellows.

Yellow is the word to define people who change your life

(a lot or a little) and whom you may or may not ever see again. It's like a new category among those who used to be called "best friends."

Most of all, there's nothing random about yellows. What I mean is that in this hypothetical airport it's perfectly possible to recognize a yellow (there are ways of recognizing them) and strike up a conversation to see if you're right, if your radar's working properly. Yellows sense each other, realize that you could be one. A relationship with a yellow doesn't begin by accident.

Haven't you ever noticed when you walk down the street that someone catches your attention? It's not necessarily a question of sexual attraction or beauty, but this person makes you feel you have to talk to him or her, to say something. It's a feeling, not love, and you suppose it can't be friendship, because friendship needs time or a job or a hobby in common. What you feel comes from seeing a yellow, being lucky enough to meet one of the yellows in your world.

What I'd like to happen is that when this book is published, someone comes up to me (or comes up to you) and says: "Would you like to be my yellow?" It would be great to be able to be like that with people. And because one of the characteristics of a yellow (although this isn't absolutely obligatory) is to be a complete stranger, it would be perfect.

But let's not get too happy. You still need to know how to find yellows, how to notice them. And know the ways (but not the rules) you need to get along with them.

Everybody knows how to get along with friends, with a partner or with a lover (although there are a thousand and one possible ways, of course). I'm going to talk about my way of dealing with yellows. In other words, what I'm going to give you is the theory, the organization, and the list, and, using that as a base, everyone can find the most appropriate way of dealing with their yellows.

Where did I get this list of how to be with yellows? Once again, from my time in the hospital. Like I said before, in the hospital you're likely to find quite a few potential yellows: Living through such an extreme situation and spending so much time together over such a short period makes it more likely for a yellow to appear.

I think that my list derives from experience, from things that we do without knowing that we do them. It's amazing, the number of things we do without knowing that we do them. A friend of mine, Eder, wrote a story where he talked about "the three seconds that we manage to look at the sun." It's true; although it is probable that nobody has ever told you that you can't look at the sun for more than three seconds, you somehow know that you can't and so you don't do it. It's strange, the sun is always above us, looking at us, heating us, and we can't bear to gaze at it for any length of time. The sun is the greatest yellow. We feel it, we notice it, we know that it's there, but we shouldn't look at it all that much.

Something similar happened in the hospital. I remember that whenever I left after being there for a long time I would say goodbye to all the people and not feel sad. I knew that they would stay there because that's where they were meant to be at that moment, and that I was going home because that's where I was meant to be. Sometimes it happened the other way around: They'd go and I would stay. I didn't feel like I was abandoning them or that I was losing them. I just felt that these roommates or these Eggheads had looked after me, listened to me, supported me, and had helped me grow. And more than anything else, that they had embraced me.

And this is how we reach another of the characteristics of the yellows, perhaps the one that most distinguishes them from friends: feeling, touching, stroking. I've never understood why we touch our friends so little—proof of the lack of evolution that there has been in friendship. Someone can be your friend and maybe never manage to come closer to you than six inches, or never give you a big hug, or never see you asleep or watch you wake up. To see how someone wakes up, how anyone wakes up, creates a sensation of closeness, of seeing someone being born, seeing them return to life; it's like a thousand, a hundred thousand conversations.

All the Eggheads, when we were in the hospital, sleeping next to one another, saw each other wake up a lot. They saw me wake up; I saw them wake up. Nobody should have to wait for a trip or an illness to see how someone sleeps and wakes up. It's something you can look for. The important thing to remember is that yellows are not just friends; friendship has very little feeling in it, very little touching, very little stroking.

I think that in friendship talking is overrated and touching is underrated; the physical distance that separates two friends isn't thought about enough.

I've always thought that it's unfair that your partner should get 95 percent of all your physical contact. Nobody would put 95 percent of their money in a single bank, but you put 95 percent of your caresses, of your hugs, into a sin-

gle person. This is where mistakes are born. This is why
there are so many infidelities. This is why people feel so
alone; this is why you notice a lack of physical contact, of
affection, of caresses.

Now that we've got to this point the question has to be
asked: Can you have sex with a yellow? And another question is also going through your head: If we're talking about
yellows, do we mean men or women?

Maybe these questions are only occurring to you now, or
maybe they've been there from the first moment that I started
to talk about this concept. Be that as it may, I have to make it
clear that my reply is conditioned by what I think, by the way
in which I have found and cultivated my yellows.

Yellows are defined by affection, stroking, and hugging.
When I talk about sleeping together and waking up together,
I'm talking about loss (sleep) and waking up (rebirth); I'm
not talking about sex. It isn't convenient to have sex with a
yellow. Of course you could, but I think that the important
thing about a yellow, about the concept of yellowness, about
the essence of yellowhood, is that yellows occupy space that
had previously been taken up by friendship. They get 40 percent physical contact, whereas beforehand friends got only
maybe 3 percent.

Now that we're here, I think it might be a good idea to
redefine yellows.

Yellow: A person who is special in your life. Yellows are
found among your friends and lovers. It's not necessary to see them regularly or keep in touch with them.
Relationships between yellows are based on affection,

stroking, and hugging. They have privileges that previously were the unique possession of a partner.

I will try to make a list of things that can be done with a yellow. The list, like everything in this book, needn't be obeyed, still less followed slavishly. Of course, each person has to decide what works and does not work for him. It's not a philosophy, it's not a religion; it's just lessons from cancer applied to life, and that's how it should be understood. So there's not really any room for debate. I know that someone's going to say: "You can sleep with a yellow." Someone else will think: "Yellows are your life partners." Another person would say: "All this nonsense about yellows doesn't make any sense. I've always had friends that I've done all this stuff with that you say you've got to do with your yellows." My response to all this: "That's fine, great." Everyone has their own friends and their own way of dealing with them. Like one of the hospital psychologists said: "Luck means being just the way you are. The shame of it is that you can't understand what other people are like."

Let's carry on, but first I need to answer the question about whether yellows are male or female. You can have girl yellows and boy yellows; what matters is the concept of yellowness, something that encompasses both sexes.

Back to the question of what you can or can't do with a yellow, which I'm sure you want to know. Here's a four-point list. We'll add more as we go on.

I should make it clear that they're not in any order, nor do you have to do all these things with a yellow. The important thing about yellows is having the feeling of having met a fellow soul, a person who marks you (an evolution in friend-ship).

After you've convinced yourself that someone can be a yellow, you can try these things with them:

1. Speaking

In this, yellows aren't much different from other kinds of re-lationships. Perhaps there's a slight difference if you're speaking to someone you don't know and what made you start speaking was the suspicion that this person was a yel-low.

With yellows you feel that you can tell them hidden se-crets, you can open yourself up. You can call them at any hour of the day or night. You feel that sometimes you don't need to maintain contact; you can spend months and months without saying anything and when you see them again every-thing is just as it always has been.

Words are overrated; it's not their quantity but their in-tensity that matters. There are yellows who are good for two conversations and yellows who are good for fifty.

2. Hugging and Stroking

This world would work better if there were more hugging and stroking. In the hospital we supported each other, we hugged each other. (The first thing you lose when you get ill is the hugs; people swap them for pats on the back. Sometimes we thought that we wouldn't die of cancer but of being patted so much on the back.)

A yellow hug lasts about two minutes. You feel the other person's breathing. It's important to feel their breathing.

As far as the stroking is concerned: Where to stroke? Wherever you want. On the hand, on the face, on the arm, on the ear, on the leg. Wherever you think you should stroke. I think it's one of the great mistakes we make, not to stroke each other more often, to feel the warmth of a hand, the temperature and touch of a hand on you.

I remember in the hospital we used to stroke each other. It was something natural, normal. It was simply and purely affection; there was no other connotation attached to it.

I think that in this particular aspect of things, yellows take on a role that has always been that of the partner. But there's no point being scared or jealous or even in thinking that you'll be misunderstood; all you have to do is change the way you think about things. Like I said before, the brain needs the right combination to let new ideas come in. You have to understand something before you judge it.

Stroking and hugging are two things that friendship doesn't include, although it's the natural next step for friends. Yellows have taken this step and enjoy its results.

3. Sleeping and Waking

Half of a yellow life is watching someone wake up. You don't have to be in the same bed, you could be in two beds, but you have to get into an environment where yellows can sleep and wake up with each other after seven or eight hours. How many people have you slept with in your life without having sex with them? Was it on a journey? Ask yourself these questions. I'm sure there won't be that many. And if you narrow it down to the people you've shared a bed with, I'm sure it'll be even fewer. This is another error that society makes: thinking that sleeping and waking are something functional, when they're actually something as important as lunch or tea.

Everyone eats with their friends. Want to have lunch? Want to come around for tea? It's something friends do. That and going on trips together. But, shall we sleep together? Hey, why not wake up together? It's not normal, but it's absolutely necessary. I'd say more: It's vital.

People think that sleeping is something so personal that it needs to be solitary or else shared via sex, but that's another area where the yellows win.

4. Separating

You should know that a yellow doesn't need as much time as a friend; you don't need to keep a yellow all your life. A yellow can be for a few hours, a few days, weeks, or years. All the time you need.

But you don't have to cultivate your yellows; you don't owe them anything, you don't need to do things for them. They have an expiration date, and they should have one. You don't even need to send a yellow an email or a text or give them a ring in order to keep something alive.

They were with you; they helped you at a particular moment or you helped them at a particular moment. Then they carried on with their journey and became yellows for other people.

Not feeling obliged to do anything is fundamental for the yellow world. Obligations, expectations: These ruin everything.

Are there yellows that last a whole lifetime? Of course there are. I have a yellow whom I've known since I was nineteen; we've spent fourteen yellow years together. He's my oldest yellow and I think we've got a few years left.

Are there yellows that only last a few hours? Yes, there are those as well. They're the ones you meet at the outpatients' clinic in a hospital, in a café, in an airport, in the street, in a swimming pool. Yellows who last hours. While I was in the hospital I managed to do all of the four things I've just listed with a lot of the people there: I had lots of roommates I slept and woke up with, whom I hugged (when we needed it), whom I spoke to about everything (death, loss, movies), and whom I lost but didn't feel sad about losing. Because what I learned from the yellows, what they said to me, continues somewhere inside me.

But lots of these people weren't yellows. I think that while I was in the hospital I got to know only seven yellows. The rest were friends.

I know that you're going to ask me how to tell the difference and, above all, how to find them. How do you go looking for them? How can you know who's a yellow and who's a friend? Well, like everything in this life, it depends a lot on each individual's sensibilities, but in the next chapter I'll give a few hints about how to answer these questions and many more.

Often, for me as a writer and for you as a reader as well, I suppose, we need a chapter to end. Sometimes it's so that we can go to sleep (some of you will be in bed already); sometimes it's so that we can leave the side of a pool, or a beach, or a hammock, or a chair, or a sofa. I hope and wish that this sofa, chair, or hammock is your favorite place to read.

Stephen King said you need to find the best place in your house to write a novel because you'll want the reader to be in the best place in his house to read it. This is how total communication is created. I can assure you that I'm in my favorite chair, writing on a screen that I've chosen for this particular occasion, and feeling very happy to be telling you all of this.

Of course, I also need this chapter to end. Writers need to finish a chapter so that they can think, reflect on what they've just written, and have a break. Just as you are about to go to sleep, or to the pool or the beach, or to go and buy bread or to meet someone who could, with luck, turn out to be a yellow.

How Do You Find Yellows and How Do You Identify Them?

How indeed? This is one of the big questions. How do you know if someone is your yellow? How do you identify them, how do you know what they are?

There's no single way; there are loads. I'm going to explain to you the theory that's the basis of the yellow world, because lots of times you need to show something and then explain where it comes from. I've already spoken a bit about the yellows, a parenthesis between "Beginning" and "Dying," but in this section on "Living" I've decided that everything's going to have to do with the yellows.

I think that there are yellows in the world so that you can find out what it is that you lack, in order to open you up and help other people open up. I'm sure that I managed to get better when I was in the hospital thanks to the seven yellows I met there. Yellows give you strength to keep fighting.

As you can see, I'm not talking about spiritual peace and harmony; I'm talking about strength to fight. There's nothing religious or cultish about yellows. Get rid of any ideas you might have in connection with those things. Yellows help us in good times or difficult times, but they are individuals. Our yellows don't form part of any collective; there's not a new yellow religion, no yellow cult, not even a worldwide yellow club.

Everybody has to be capable of looking for yellows when they need them, but not in the sense that they need to rush out into the street looking like crazy for yellows. Yellows will appear; you'll run into them when you need them.

But everyone has only twenty-three yellows. I know twenty-three seems like a small number, but it's the right number. I've always believed in the power of twenty-three; it's the magic number. Blood takes twenty-three seconds to travel around the human body; the spinal column has twenty-three discs; they stabbed Julius Caesar twenty-three times. Sex is described in chromosome twenty-three, and each man and woman gives twenty-three chromosomes to their child.

In fact, twenty-three's amazing. But it's not just these facts that make me think that twenty-three is something basic in life, it's because I've got a personal relationship with the number: I lost my leg on April 23. And I started to think that it was true what a lot of people said, that twenty-three is connected with lots of people's lives, and that if you are looking for an exact number for anything in this world it's bound to be twenty-three. It's a number loved by nature.

So I believe in this number, in its positive potential. I'm completely convinced that twenty-three is a magical number, a lucky number. Curiously, there are also twenty-three discoveries in this book.

So let's carry on with this premise that you have only

twenty-three yellows in this world. How do you find them? Should you look for them very slowly so that they last you your whole life?

The answer for how to look for them depends on you as an individual. You should look for them when you need them. How you find them depends on what I call marks.

Marks, or traces, are the way you recognize a yellow. Here's an example: I've got a great friend who lives in Colombia, in Cali. I've never been to Colombia; he's never been to Barcelona. But six years ago we met each other on a chat site for cripples; he was missing a leg and so was I. I think that someone wanted us to meet each other, marked us, and set us down in two places on the earth. The way that we got to know each other was this mark, which was like a coincidence, a chance, a signal that we had to meet. When I say "someone" I don't mean God or any kind of being; I mean nature, the natural order of things.

It's the same with the yellows: Someone has marked twenty-three yellows for you to meet them. So you have to make the effort to find what your marks are, because they're not the same for everyone.

I could leave it here, like one of those secrets that you don't tell anyone. M. Night Shyamalan, the director of *The Sixth Sense*, was speaking in Barcelona a while back, and he said that he was going to tell us a secret, something that no one knew and that he was going to trust to us. We all drew closer, listened to him with our full attention. He wanted to tell us the secret of his success, how he made *The Sixth Sense*, and why, after two failures, he'd known that his third film would be a success.

The whole auditorium was on edge; we wanted to hear the secret. And he said: "I decided to watch films by directors who have only ever had one hit in their lives. I saw a lot of these films and found eight common denominators, which I used to make *The Sixth Sense*."

That was it. I'm not lying. It was a secret that left you wondering, and I can't think of anything worse than that. Everyone felt cheated; when someone tells you a secret it shouldn't leave you in the dark. But maybe that's what M. Night Shyamalan wanted. I started watching the films he recommended and came to my own eight conclusions, but I don't know if they were his or not. But actually, as time went by, I realized I'm glad he didn't tell us what they were, because we'd only have copied him and repeated him. Everyone has to find their own common denominators, come to their own conclusions.

So I'll tell you the way to find your marks, but then it has to be you who makes finding them a reality. So that it's something tangible.

Everything to do with finding yellows has to do with beauty. I've always believed that beauty is something senseless, chaotic. What one person finds beautiful another person will think is horrible. Beauty is relative. Why are people attracted by a particular head shape, body type, way of speaking, way of looking, way of not looking? I've never understood it. It's something that fascinates me. You can be in a room with five thousand other people and you can say which are the beautiful ones, which ones are beautiful according to your criteria. But this beauty has different aspects: poetical beauty, sexual beauty, yellow beauty.

Beauty is something the yellow mark hides behind. Hasn't it ever happened that you see a figure in a crowd and you just can't take your eyes off them? It's got nothing to do with sex, you don't want to sleep with this person; it's just that they fill a gap in your world. You think that they understand you, that you could be friends, that there's a common energy between you. Then the person disappears and you forget about them. They won't stay long in your memory; it's as if their departure caused no sadness, it was something that had to be accepted. This is part of the yellow world; yellows leave and don't make you sad. And this happens even if you don't know them.

The most important thing is to be able to distinguish between things, to take from beauty all the signs that have something to do with the yellows.

How to do it? I'll tell you my method, the one I use to find the marks of my yellows. Although they won't all work for you, each day more of them will be successful. You'll note them down, corroborate them, and, above all, apply them to the yellows you already have. This helps prove that they are marks.

In list form, the method is as follows:

1. You need to try to understand what beauty is for you. Find your own criteria of beauty and note them down. They need to be connected with people who grab your attention as soon as you look at them.

   They don't have to be only adjectives: They can be sounds, colors, objects, everything you think is beautiful.

There are thousands of examples. If beauty has something to do with white towels, write it down. If it's a kind of haircut, write it down. If it's the smell of a corduroy jacket, write it down. If it's what eyes and a mouth look like inside a motorcycle helmet, write it down. Maybe you've hit upon something so strange it really is a yellow mark. Yellow marks tend to be complicated and recherché.

2. Once you've got the list, which, to work properly, needs to have a hundred entries, start to get rid of everything that's got something to do with the beauties of sex and love.

Let me explain. Anything that's got anything to do with sex or love doesn't count. I'm sure you've written down how important the shape of someone's lips is, but that's bound to have some kind of sexual connotation; it's nothing to do with yellow beauty, only with sexual beauty.

But you have to be careful, because sometimes you could get rid of a characteristic that seems sexual but is in fact yellow. These things happen, but what you have to do is accept the mistake, because sooner or later you'll realize you've overlooked something.

This isn't a science; there's no point driving yourself crazy putting criteria in and crossing them out; you should enjoy the search. You have to enjoy yourself because there's no such thing as absolute truth, only relative truths. Mistakes are possible and you have to accept them.

I'm sure that, out of a list of a hundred, you'll get

rid of about seventy-seven that have something to do with the beauties of sex and love, and so there'll be twenty-three left.

3. Twenty-three again, I know. Well, these twenty-three beauty points that you haven't been able to get rid of, these twenty-three things that you don't know why but which seem beautiful to you, are what we'll start working with. You have to have your radar turned on, and when you find at least three of these points in a person, you'll know that there's an outside chance that he or she's a yellow. If it's nine the possibility stops being remote and becomes a likelihood. If it's more than thirteen you have to speak to this person, because they're bound to be a yellow. If you get the whole twenty-three, bingo, there you go. You can let them escape if you don't need them at that moment or else speak to that person if you want to or see that you need to. What you have to remember is that it's one thing to meet a yellow and another to speak with them. Remember: You will find them, but you mustn't waste them. There aren't a lot of them and they do have an expiration date. So it's up to you.

4. And if you do decide to speak to this person, what then? You'll start a yellow relationship that will last as long as it needs to last; it could be hours, or months, or years. And when it finishes you'll feel better, but you'll also feel changed. And when you've changed, your marks will change, your insides will change.

5. And so, every two years, more or less, you need to look for your marks again. Every two years yellow beauty

changes, thanks to contact with a yellow. So look for your marks every couple of years. You'll find that fifteen or sixteen will have stayed the same, but seven or eight will have changed. It's important to work out what they are so you don't make a mistake.

I know that it's a difficult task, and that now you're starting to have doubts. Are these the signs of yellow beauty, or the beauties of sex and love?

The best way to find out is to collect photos that catch your attention: photos of people in newspapers and magazines, pictures from the Internet. Languages with accents that attract you. Smells that you can't get out of your head and that seem beautiful to you. Images that have stuck in your memory.

In your mind you have to run through everything that seems beautiful. Don't think only about people but also places, periods of your life, feelings, and sensations. You'll have to do a lot of searching.

But it's just what M. Night Shyamalan said: To understand the secret you need to work a lot. But it's worth it. You have to work, but the yellow world is worth it.

I know that maybe some ideas aren't clear to you. So in the next chapter I'll give you a yellow Q&A, which I hope will help to sort out whatever's going around in your head.

Yellow Q&A

I like computers. For some reason, I get along well with them. I like knowing that when things don't work you can turn the computer off and on again; it's a magical solution.

I think it wouldn't be a bad idea if we could do the same with people, so when you didn't understand someone or when someone behaved strangely you could reboot them, turn them off and on again.

This is the first thing that I'd bring to our world; the next would be the "undo" button that you get on computers. It's amazing. If you make a mistake and click on undo, a little arrow rotates, then you get back the last thing you've done.

I don't know how many times a day I click undo. I'm sure it must be an average of one or two hundred times a day. We never think we've made the right decision.

And what if we could undo things in our lives? I'm sure that loads of people would go back to when they were twenty and avoid doing something, or when they were fifteen and not do another, or when they were eight. . . . Maybe even go back to when they were born, and not be born.

The third thing I like about computers is the "help" tab that programs have. There must be things that confuse a lot of people, and the programmers, who know this, include the answers in the program itself. I like it when I find my problem in the help database, because I know then that it's going to be solved. But, do you know what? I also like it when my problem isn't in the database, because it shows that I'm not as predictable as they think I am. I like that my problems are strange, surprising, and, most of all, new. It makes me feel alive.

So don't worry if your problem isn't in the yellow Q&A. It means you're alive, really alive. And I'm sure you'll find the answer somewhere.

Can a family member be a yellow?

Of course they can. Our brothers and sisters are the first possible yellows, prime candidates for yellowhood. You've slept with them if you shared a room when you were little. They hug you and stroke you. They are, or can be, yellows.

Fathers and mothers can also be yellows, but it's less likely. But I am sure that cases exist.

You have to remember that anyone can be a yellow.

Can yellows become friends, or lovers, or sexual partners?

In life everything can change. I call it getting paler or getting brighter. Sometimes they become a paler yellow and turn into friends. Sometimes they go a bit orangey and become lovers, people you love.

You and your yellow need to decide what it is you want to be. What is sure is that there's no way back. When the yellow becomes brighter or paler, there's no way back to being yellow.

So think it through first.

What happens if I find out that someone is my yellow, but the person doesn't believe in yellows? Should I tell them?

Well, it takes two to yellow. I mean that someone can be your yellow only if you are their yellow. It's not possible for someone to be your yellow and for you to mean nothing to them; it's a two-way relationship.

I said that this wouldn't be easy. It might also happen that someone doesn't want to be your yellow (because they don't believe in yellows or don't think of you as a yellow); in that case you have to let them go, forget about them. Maybe it wasn't the right moment to have that yellow.

In life you have to know how to say no and accept it when other people say no. Other opportunities will arise. Anyway, who knows? Maybe you made a mistake and they weren't a yellow.

What do I talk about with a yellow?

I haven't wanted to discuss this topic beforehand because I think that everyone should talk about whatever they want with their yellows. It doesn't have to be deep things; they can be banal conversations that make you feel good.

The purpose of finding a yellow isn't to have complicated conversations that will change the world, or your world, but for these people to give some sort of meaning to your world. They calm your inner struggle; they give you peace.

I also didn't want to talk about this very much so as not to condition you, make you think that you have to talk about a particular topic. Topics will arise, don't you worry. The yellows bring them with themselves.

I think that everyone has their circle of people they can talk to, who make them feel good, who have something special that ties them together. These are friends who should be turned into yellows right away.

If I'm a boy, will I have more yellows who are boys or more yellows who are girls?

It has nothing to do with sex; not everything in life has to do with sex. I imagine you'll have boy yellows and girl yellows. The beauty we've been talking about has nothing to do with your sexuality but with details and marks that appear and that you can't understand at first sight.

There'll be a bit of everything, like there is at each age as you grow up: There's no fixed rule.

(Although there are always exceptions.) You don't have to think about rules; think about lists.

What if someone pretends to be my yellow but only wants to be stroked or hugged or to sleep with me?

Whenever you think of a concept, someone else perverts it, or uses it, or changes it. It is we who will use the concept of yellowness and we who should know how to use it.

So the answer is that if you discover such a thing, you'll realize it stands against everything that the concept of yellowness stands for, and you'll know what to do.

What if I don't know how to make the list? What if I don't have any yellows? Is that possible?

Maybe where you're at right now you don't need yellows, and if you don't need them then maybe you won't find the marks. Give yourself time—it's not something that you'll get done in half an hour; it might even take you a whole year.

What are your marks?

I think that everyone should keep his marks secret, which is why I haven't said what mine are. I don't think you should make them public. It's as if that would make them lose a bit of their value. When you've gone to all the trouble of finding out what the marks are, then you should know how to value this effort. And it should be *your* effort, your own personal and private effort.

You could tell them to another yellow if you need to, but I don't think you should need to.

Do you have to tell someone you want to be their yellow, or can you simply get to know them without revealing that they're your yellow?

You don't always have to ask someone if they want to be your yellow. You can carry on like you've been doing for the time being—meeting yellows and not seeing them again—but the good thing is that you'll now know that those people were yellows. You'll be calmer and feel happier.

Can you introduce two yellows to each other? Can they be each other's yellows?

There's no point: The nine or ten marks that made you think that a particular person was a yellow won't be the same ones that made the other person think that they were your yellow.

Of course you can introduce two yellows, that'd be great, but it doesn't mean that they'll be each other's yellows.

What about friends? Are they now second-class citizens?

Far from it. Friends are there, but some of them evolve and turn into yellows. It's just another rung on the ladder.

Here's a list of relationships. The order doesn't mean that any one is better than another.

1. Acquaintances: people you meet once at work, or in the street, who introduce themselves but whom you're not quite in tune with yet.
2. Friends: These can be from school, from work, from college, from a hobby in common. They're people you like, whom you feel a connection with, whom you have fun with, who help you, who tell you things, and whom you can hug and stroke and sleep next to. If that's what you feel like. Maybe they're not yellows, but that doesn't mean you can't treat them like yellows.
3. Yellows: Everyone has twenty-three of them, and they are something more than friends. They're people you meet and who change your life (either in the short or the long term). Exchange affection, hugs, stroking; sleep next to them. They help your life balance out; they stop your partner having a monopoly on you. Yellows get 40 percent of all physical contact.
4. Partners or lovers: They still exist, nothing changes,

but they no longer have a monopoly on physical contact. They have to learn how to share and know that the yellows get a 40 percent share. This doesn't mean that your partner loses 40 percent but that you now get 135 percent physical contact.

In my ideal world the best thing would be to transform your friends into yellows, to overcome the twenty-three barrier.

What if my partner doesn't understand about the yellows?

All types of change are complicated. Jealousy is something natural. How can the person you love understand that you're sleeping with other people? Only by understanding the concept, understanding that in the yellow world you need to see your fellow yellows sleep and wake up.

I know that I could write a hundred questions here. But manuals of instruction always have twelve, the twelve most important questions. So, like I said, if your question isn't here then rejoice—it's not one of the typical ones, it's something new.

Conclusions About Yellows

"Living" is coming to its end. . . . This is a brief summary of the things you have to do to find your yellows. A little list to guide you into this new world, this new step in your friendships, this new way of understanding the world.

Do it. Change your world.

Make a list of the yellows you think you have had

First gather all the yellows. Without knowing it, you'll have had five or six before now who you didn't know were yellows. Put them in a list. You don't need to ask them; they were and are yellows. You can even call them and tell them.

Look for your yellow marks

Think about the word *beauty* and make a list of marks. Get rid of all the ones that are marks of sex or of love. This list is the basis for everything.

Use photos, pictures, smells, and even the list of yellows you've already got. They will surely be the basis for your yellow marks.

Look for yellows and let them find you

Search for your yellows. You can find them at work, in the street, in a train station. Let them in and enter into them as well.

All you need is a single question: Do you want to be my yellow?

Enjoy your yellows

The most important thing is conversation. You'll see how everything flows so smoothly, as if they are open to you and you are open to them.

Let yourself be filled with the essence of yellowness. And above all go for physical contact, without fear, without jealousy, without any type of shame.

Lose them, keep them, renew them

It depends on you. They could be yellows for your whole life long, or they could turn into friends, into lovers, into whatever you want.

And remember, it's the yellows who renew you. They change you, so every couple of years try to go back and look for your marks again.

Above all, enjoy yourself. This is the basis. Enjoyment.

How better to finish than with a new definition of yellow?

Yellow: A special person in our life, whom we stroke, hug, and sleep next to. They mark our lives, and the relationship with them doesn't take time or effort. There are twenty-three in our lives. Conversations with them make us better people and help us discover what we are lacking. They are the next level of friendship.

And Relax . . .

The Yellow End

Don't be so crazy. Best behavior. Stand up straight.
Don't drink. Don't smoke. Don't cough. Don't breathe.
Yes, don't breathe! Say no to every "no"
And relax: die.

—Gabriel Celaya

The Yellow End

Although I've focused on life, I have to end, like Celaya did, with death.

This was another lesson I learned from cancer. I lost my fear of death and this is something I thought I would forget about when I started to live without cancer, but in fact just the opposite happened. I am still not afraid of death and this has a great deal to do with the years of fighting against my illness and such continuous contact with death. As I said, a lot of my friends died. But they're all close to me, and 3.7 of them I've got inside me, deep within.

At a lot of the talks that I give, people ask me how you lose your fear of death. How can you manage to do it? Do you have to have a mortal illness? What does it mean to lose your fear of death: Are you braver; are you more impulsive; have you lost your fear of everything?

People want a quick fix: Do this and you'll lose your fear of death. Quick fixes don't exist. Lists of pieces of advice exist, lists of possible things that you can do. But as with everything, you have to internalize them, believe them to be true, and, little by little, put them into practice.

In these talks I usually explain the importance of talking about death. You can't lose your fear of something if you don't talk about it. You have to believe that it's something natural, something that you'll go through, nothing negative.

Death is not bad. Death dignifies everything, gives it an end.

I have written lots of screenplays and teach screenwriting, and the first thing I tell my students is that in order to be a good screenwriter you need to know how you will end the film, how it will finish. A good ending can give you a good film. If you don't know anything about the ending, if you're scared of it, then maybe the film will never finish. Lots of times I've thought up endings that deserved a story in front of them; sometimes you find them and sometimes you don't. But you can't do anything without an end.

Life is the same. You have to speak naturally about your end. Speak of your death and the deaths of people around you.

It might seem complicated, but in fact it's quite simple; all you have to do is put it into practice. In the hospital we Egg-heads spoke a lot about death: We all knew that we might die soon and that gave us a strong desire to talk about it. To know how it would take each of us, to know how other people would like to die, to know what you thought about your death.

I feel my heart start to beat more strongly when I talk about this—this is a good sign. You shouldn't confuse emotion with sadness. I feel emotion; it makes me happy to think about those kids who died. I've never felt pity or sadness for them; they didn't deserve it, they didn't deserve for their memory to be connected with either of those two feelings.

There are people who tell me that it's not easy to ask someone how they want to die or how they want to be remembered. I always tell them that the best thing is to start at a distance and get closer by degrees. I like asking new friends this question: Which death has affected you the most?

Just this question about death opens up paths, you discover so many things. . . . People are happy to talk about jobs they're going to do, girlfriends they're going to have, or journeys they're going to take. And maybe they won't go on those journeys, maybe they won't get those girls, maybe they won't get those jobs. But they'll definitely die.

Talking about the death that has hurt you the most is most likely to make you talk about a death that you haven't yet overcome. The most painful deaths are the ones that haven't been accepted, the ones that are remembered the most.

What should you do if someone tells you about a death that hasn't yet been overcome? Just listen, ask lots of questions, and nothing else. It's almost as if they are telling you about a journey or a new experience. And above all, don't feel pity for them. How absurd pity is! It's completely useless.

I think that death marks you in a way that life cannot. There are people whose father or mother died when they were little. These kids talk about their father or mother in a special way; they have been marked and they have had to do things that otherwise they wouldn't have done. Death is important for the legacies it leaves; it adds the finishing touch to things.

You always have to think of death as something good. People celebrate life, celebrate baptisms; they should celebrate deaths like this as well. It would be a part of the memory, of the dignification of the deceased.

I know some people think that I'm being frivolous about death when I say that it's something good, because surely they've been through the painful death of loved ones and don't find anything beautiful in it. But what you have to remember is that in itself death doesn't exist. When someone dies they turn into someone you have known. Memories of them remain; their life is divided among the people who knew them. It's as if they were being multiplied in lots of people.

Don't connect death with pain. Don't connect death with loss. Connect it to life, connect it to a dignified end. Don't think that you're going to disappear, don't be afraid of disappearing. It's something that you'll do sooner or later.

I think that the more you speak to your friends and family about your own death the more prepared everyone will be. I'm not talking about making a will, just simply asking people to do things you'd like them to do when you die. In the hospital the Eggheads wanted a huge number of things; for example, one of us wanted, when he was dead, for all the rest of us to go to a concert in New York. Desires from beyond death, beautiful wishes that I've tried to carry out. Wishes that were full of life.

When I wrote María Ripoll's film *Your Life in 65 Minutes* I went maybe even further. The film was about a kid who was so happy that he didn't want to continue; he wanted to put a proper ending to things. It wasn't an apologia for suicide, but a film about life and death. Why can't you want to die in the same way that lots of people want to live? Why should you always want more if you've got everything in life, if you've reached the heights of happiness? These were the premises of the film. Sometimes you have to go to extremes in order to make people get centered.

I would like to die on a Friday. I like Fridays; it's when the new releases come out in the cinema and people are usually happy. I liked Fridays a lot when I was little because my parents would come to school to pick me up, give me a tuna sandwich, and take me to Cardedeu, where we had a summer house. We always got stuck in traffic jams on the way and my father would always put the radio on; this is where I heard the first songs that really excited me. I remember most clearly when I first heard Stevie Wonder's "I Just Called to Say I Love You." It made me stop eating my tuna sandwich. It seemed so beautiful that I was transfixed while the trumpets and the violins mingled with the clicking of the turn signal.

I'd like to die on Friday because such beautiful things happen on Fridays!

You should start by asking for a date of death: a day, a season, a place. It's nothing creepy; death isn't creepy; leaving this world isn't creepy. In fact, thinking about your death is necessary and should be obligatory. They should teach "life and death" in schools. No black humor—it would be fun, and it's important for us to have contact with the end of our lives from the time we are children. That great book

Tuesdays with Morrie tells us that "learning to die helps you learn to live." I want to go further: Think about your death, think about the details, think about the end, and you'll be able to think about your life, concrete ideas about what you want to do in this world.

Death is something fundamental in the yellow world. The yellow world is based on knowing what you can lose and what you can win. Life is about that: losing and winning. There'll be times when you only lose, so remember that there was a time when all you did was win.

To finish this chapter off, here's a little list about death:

1. Think about death as something positive.

2. Talk with your friends about their deaths or deaths that have affected them. Let the conversation flow; forget about pity and that you are talking about a taboo topic.

3. When someone dies and you go to the funeral, don't try to avoid talking about it. Forget the phrases "My thoughts are with you," "I'm sorry for your loss." Look for the phrases that truly define the death. There is no set phrase for a death, but don't use a phrase that says nothing. It has to come out of you. It could be a detail from the dead person's life, maybe what you felt when you heard about the death.

4. Call your friends and family after the death of a loved one. Don't be afraid. Call after twenty-four hours, ask questions, talk about what they're feeling, and keep on doing this for as long as you think necessary. It's bound to be one of the things that have marked them most in

their life. Why do you think they'd be upset talking about something so important?

5. Think about your own death. Think about the day, the season, what the weather should be like, the place, who you'd like to be with. Don't think about whether you'd like to be buried or cremated. Think about the moment—nothing but the moment—not what happens afterward.

6. Talk with your friends about these details. And explain to them the things you'd like them to do after your death, things filled with life. Not things to do on the anniversary of your death or in the cemetery, but things that celebrate life. There was one Egghead who said that if he died one day and I wrote a book, he'd like the word *grapefruit* to appear somewhere in it. He loved grapefruit, thought it was the best fruit in the world. I said I would put it in. He died a year later. Now when I see the word *grapefruit* written down I feel that he's alive, he's fine, and he's inside me. I can imagine his face, his eyes; I see the grapefruit being eaten. Can someone who makes us feel so much actually be dead?

7. Die. Whenever, whenever it's your turn. Don't look for death but don't be scared of it, either. Cancer made me bump up against death lots of times. Meet it head-on. And forget your fears: fear of losing your friends, fear of losing things, fear of losing who you are. You don't actually lose anything, nothing at all. Believe me, stand back from the fear, stand back from the terror, and look the word *death* in the face. Visualize it. Nothing else.

Epilogue

It's over.

I feel good.

I like what I've written; I hope you like reading it.

These last words complete the journey of my Egghead memories onto these pages.

Thank you, Eloy, for the great Afterword. I've just gotten it and it touched me; it hit me right in the esophagus. You make me happy.

I see how thick the book will be and the color it'll have. I thought that it could flow and it did flow.

Nothing else, I'll leave you now. And I hope that you'll meet me.

And remember: Trust your dreams and they'll come true.

Afterword

"Careful, this book is Albert. If you get into it you won't want to get out."

Albert has the curiosity of Sherlock Holmes and the looks of Dr. Watson. He's so scruffy it makes you wonder if he spends time making himself look scruffy before he leaves his house. He's so weird that it's even attractive.

One of his favorite activities is looking. Without permission, he enters your head through your eyes and gets all the information he needs. His emotional radar is almost infallible and judges people as easily as those supermarket checkouts that know how much your goods cost simply by reading the bar code. When he's right he knows more about you than you do yourself.

Albert has won several battles with death, which is why his stories are so full of life. He's hyperactive, and prefers losing sleep to losing experiences. His mind works so fast that it makes you dizzy. If you want to tell him something it has to be very good or told very fast.

If you want to catch his interest, don't tell him about your life; let him find out about it for himself. This is another of his favorite activities.

He loves to provoke people but he does it in order to make provocations normal. He gave me an audition for his film *Don't Ask Me to Kiss You, Because I Will Kiss You,* where we practiced a sequence in an imaginary swimming pool. I'd just met him. Suddenly he took off his artificial leg. He did this so normally that I touched my leg to see if I could do the same. It was a hysterical action on my part—I was trying to appear normal—but this really knocked me off my stride. He realized this, and with the same normality that he had removed his left leg he started to talk to me about one of the most recurrent themes in his life and his movies: the world of masturbation. We formed an immediate connection. I forgot the audition, forgot about the leg, forgot that he was the director, and found myself next to a guy who was talking about feelings we all share.

He looks thirty, but he's spent more than fifteen years recovering his adolescence. This is how he can be so fresh and so clean. This is how he can keep on thinking about whatever he can imagine, everything he can do.

Albert is powerful because he never gives up. And as a last resort he bargains: He swapped a leg and a lung for his life. He has learned how to lose in order to win. And he writes: plays, films, TV series, novels . . . He uses humor to show us human drama. And he connects daily reality with our most distant dreams. And now he wants to tell you that the only handicaps are emotional, that we live in a society that doesn't value feelings.

Albert wants to tell us about a world that's within everyone's reach, a world the color of the sun: the yellow world. A warm place where kisses can last ten minutes, where strangers can be your greatest helpers, where physical contact loses its sexual overtones, where receiving affection is something as basic as buying bread, where fear has no meaning, where death isn't just something that happens to other people, where life is the most important thing, where everything is wherever you want it to be.

This book tells us about all of this, everything that we feel and we don't say, about the fear that they'll take what we have away from us, about being able to recognize ourselves in our entirety and appreciate who we are every second of the day. Long live Albert!

—Eloy Azorín, actor

About the Author

ALBERT ESPINOSA is an industrial engineer, screenwriter, actor, and director. He is the creator of the hit Catalan television series *Polseres vermelles* (known in English as *Red Band Society*) and the author of three novels. He has written screenplays for the internationally acclaimed films *Your Life in 65 Minutes,* *Nobody's Perfect,* and *4th Floor.* He debuted as a film director in 2007 with *No me pidas que te bese porque te besaré,* which he also wrote and starred in himself.

www.albertespinosa.com
@espinosa_albert
Facebook.com/Albert.Espinosa.Oficial

About the Type

This book was set in Sabon, a typeface designed by the well-known German typographer Jan Tschichold (1902–74). Sabon's design is based upon the original letter forms of sixteenth-century French type designer Claude Garamond and was created specifically to be used for three sources: foundry type for hand composition, Linotype, and Monotype. Tschichold named his typeface for the famous Frankfurt typefounder Jacques Sabon (c. 1520–80).